LEGAL FRONTIERS

—— OF ——

DEATH AND DYING

Medical Ethics series
David H. Smith and Robert M. Veatch, editors

LEGAL FRONTIERS

—— OF ——

DEATH AND DYING

BY

NORMAN L. CANTOR

INDIANA UNIVERSITY PRESS
BLOOMINGTON AND INDIANAPOLIS

For Tamar

Manufactured in the United States of America
Library of Congress Cataloging-in-Publication Data

Cantor, Norman L.
  Legal frontiers of death and dying.

  (Medical ethics series)
  Includes index.
    1. Terminal care—Law and legislation—United States.
  2. Death—Proof and certification—United States.
    3. Right to die—Law and legislation—United States.
  I. Title. II. Series.
  KF3827.E87C36 1987   344.73'0419   86-45502
  ISBN 0-253-33290-7   347.304419

1 2 3 4 5 91 90 89 88 87

CONTENTS

ACKNOWLEDGMENTS

Because most of this book was written in Tel Aviv, the usual coterie of typists, secretaries, research assistants, etc., was lacking. Economic austerity was a fact of life during this period in Israeli higher education. The consequence is that I must take responsibility not only for the contents, but for many of the chores of production. With all that, I did benefit from the able research assistance of Paul Zelenty, a student at Rutgers Law School, and David Grossman, formerly a student there and now an attorney. I thank Dean Peter Simmons of Rutgers and Dean Uri Reichmann of Tel Aviv University for their encouragement and backing. Finally, I thank Assistant Dean Linda Garbaccio for considerable administrative assistance despite the difficulties and frustrations of trans-Atlantic communications.

INTRODUCTION

Modern medical technology has made it possible to keep patients "alive" longer and longer—sometimes beyond the point dictated by humane medical practice. Beginning in the early 1960s, this fact prompted considerable soul searching by medical practitioners and commentators on the medical scene. Their principal concern was the easing of suffering for some terminally ill patients. The threshold question was whether it was ever legally permissible to withhold or withdraw life-preserving care from a medical patient. For the common assumption had been that preservation of life was a preeminent value, and that legal and ethical constraints mandated every effort to keep a patient alive.

A number of subissues flowed from the basic question whether life-preserving care could ever be terminated. Could a competent adult patient dictate the cessation of care and, if so, must those instructions follow some special format? Would the patient's wishes be honored after the patient had become incompetent? Was termination limited to "extraordinary" medical measures and, if so, how was that term to be defined? Was termination confined to passive withholding of medical measures, or could physicians actively terminate or disconnect procedures previously instituted?

The famous Karen Ann Quinlan case in 1976—involving a permanently comatose individual—shifted focus from the competent to the incompetent patient. The question became whether life-preserving care could legally be removed from an incompetent patient. And who could make such a determination—the patient's physician, the patient's guardian, a hospital committee, a court? According to what criteria could such a terminal decision be made? Were the patient's previously expressed wishes determinative? Must the decision-maker strive to replicate what the patient would have wanted if the patient were hypothetically competent to decide? Or must the decision-maker simply act to implement the "best interests" of the incompetent patient? If "best interests" is indeed the applicable standard, how is that term to be defined, i.e., what specific factors comprise the best interests of an incompetent patient?

Over the last twenty years, particularly during the eleven since *Quinlan* was decided, judicial authority and associated legal commentary have begun to offer guidance in the resolution of most of the above issues and subissues. Judicial sentiment is by no means unanimous. Nor are the

ix

answers available from any single source of legal authority. Death and dying issues are being resolved with a unique blend of criminal law, constitutional law, torts, contracts, professional ethics, and guardianship principles. But despite this complexity, certain trends are perceptible in both the judicial and legislative responses to the issues.

This book's primary objective is to scrutinize the legal responses to the above questions with the goal of discerning and analyzing the emerging trends. One overwhelming conclusion is that legal authorities have recognized that the important object of preserving human existence must be tempered by respect for human dignity. At the very least, this means that a terminally ill medical patient need not be sustained in a condition where existence is dominated by unrelenting physical and/or emotional pain. But human dignity in the context of death and dying is coming to mean something more—namely, respect for a human prerogative to exercise self-determination. I will consider the precise extent to which legal decisions in the context of terminal illness can and should respect the autonomy of competent adult patients.

I will also examine the status of "death with dignity" in the context of incompetent, terminally ill patients. Where patients have previously left directions as to their own future handling, this largely means respect for self-determination. But courts have gone further, to accept the notion that incompetent patients may be allowed to die once existence has reached a stage at which no interest of the patient is served by further resistance to the dying process. Again, while life is a sacrosanct value, humane handling of dying patients does not demand unrelenting preservation of every person's existence.

Establishment of these general principles has led to new issues only dimly perceived when the first inquiries were made as to whether medical patients had to be kept alive at all costs. These emerging "frontier" issues are the second focus of this book. The first group of these issues concern the prerogatives of competent patients. To what extent can a patient resist treatment for a life-threatening condition when the patient is salvageable—that is, when the patient's status could be maintained for a substantial period, or even when the patient could be returned to a healthful existence? There are two subissues here. Must death be "imminent" before a patient may invoke a right to resist life-preserving treatment? And must the patient be terminally ill—not salvageable to a healthful existence—before the wish to have care terminated will be honored? The last question has particular relevance to hunger strikers and to disabled citizens who seek to invoke a right to resist life-preserving medical treatment in order to refuse forced feeding by governmental authorities.

The remaining "frontier" issues relate to the handling of incompetent patients. In particular, hard questions surround the chronically ill, senile, elderly person whose condition deteriorates to a point where cognitive existence is barely discernible. At what point, if any, do "quality of life" considerations allow for the withdrawal of life-sustaining medical procedures from such persons? As to the general class of incompetent patients, further "frontier" issues exist. Can the interests of parties other than the patient—for example, economic and emotional concerns of family—play a role in the decision whether to terminate life-preserving care? Can nourishment in the form of intravenous feeding or nasogastric tubes be regarded as one of the medical procedures withdrawable from patients? And when, if ever, can life-preserving care be withheld or withdrawn from defective infants? What criteria govern medical intervention for these humans with neither communication ability nor life experience which could inform a judgment as to their "best interests?" A closely related question is to what extent the commonly acknowledged interest in family autonomy insulates parental decisions to allow infants to die. Does the federal Constitution circumscribe the scope of judicial review of parental decisions in this context? And what is the appropriate role of the federal government in regulating the policies and procedures of hospitals handling neonatal cases?

As to these various "frontier issues," judicial authority is sparse. This book seeks to synthesize the legal currents emerging from opinions examining the more basic issues concerning the handling of terminal medical patients, and to indicate how the frontier questions will and should be resolved. An effort will also be made to debunk the myth that "quality of life" considerations are anathema in the death and dying context. The reality is that it is far more humane to relieve the suffering of dying patients and to honor patient self-determination, than to exalt "protection of innocent life" as an all encompassing bar to the withdrawal of life-preserving care. Nor does the injection of quality of life considerations necessarily jeopardize the status of defective newborns, mental retardates, senile persons, or other handicapped individuals. Quality of life does not mean a rational utility assessment of personal worth—an elimination of lives because they are not worthwhile, or socially useful, or because they constitute a burden on people around them. World experience with eugenic euthanasia and slavery caution against careless relegation of persons to subhuman status. This experience dictates that principled limitations be imposed on utilization of "quality of life" factors in handling medical patients. One thesis of this book is that such limitations can be found.

A disclaimer is appropriate. Throughout this book I differentiate between "competent" and "incompetent" patients. In doing so I simply gloss over the complexities involved in making determinations of which patients are in fact competent for purposes of life and death decisions. Similarly, I don't enter the thicket of "informed consent," the theoretical and applied difficulties of conveying sufficient information to patients (and/or families) to permit genuine participation in decision-making. It is not that I'm unappreciative of these problems. They are merely beyond the scope of this book.

LEGAL FRONTIERS
—————— OF ——————
DEATH AND DYING

I

DECISIONS BY COMPETENT PATIENTS

> Vex not his ghost: O, let him pass! he hates him
> That would upon the rack of this tough world
> Stretch him out longer.
>
> KING LEAR V, iii

The original rallying cry of those advocating a right to refuse life-preserving medical treatment was "death with dignity." The object was to spare pain and suffering to a terminally ill patient whose life was being unrelentingly protracted by well intentioned but overzealous medical personnel. A prolonged dying process, accompanied by physical and emotional suffering, was viewed as undignified and unnecessary in the face of approaching, unpreventable death.

The "death with dignity" movement appealed both to humane instincts and common sense. Very few persons favor suffering for its own sake. Most people understand and respect a dying person's considered opinion that, for the individual involved, pain or degradation in the dying process warrant giving up the medical struggle against impending death. Even those who believe that it's a divine prerogative to fix the timing of death understand that intervention of medical technology may cruelly and artificially prolong what would otherwise be a naturally occurring dying process.

Not surprisingly, then, in the wake of the "death with dignity" movement widespread judicial, legislative, and medical acceptance has been extended to a patient's prerogative to resist life-preserving medical treatment in the context of an immediate terminal condition. There may not be unanimity in tracing the origin of the legal right—whether it be the federal Constitution, state statutes, or judicially evolved common law doctrine—but the right is widely acknowledged to belong to a suffering,

1

terminally ill patient. More controversial is the willingness of some courts to extend the patient's prerogative to resist treatment to situations where death is not imminent, or even to situations where the patient can be entirely restored to a healthy existence. These extensions will be examined below after attention is given to the clearer case of the suffering patient facing an imminent and certain demise.

Patients Facing Unavoidable, Imminent Death

The theme of avoiding unnecessary suffering is so well accepted that few cases are litigated in which medical personnel question the prerogative of a competent, dying patient to resist continued medical intervention. Judicial attention is more often drawn to the handling of incompetent patients—and in that context, courts start with the premise that a competent, dying patient is entitled to resist continued treatment. The judges then move from that premise to resolve the status of the incompetent patient, a subject which will be addressed in chapter 3.

Satz v. Perlmutter,[1] a 1979 Florida case, represents one of the few instances when the wishes of a hopelessly ill, competent patient were contested all the way to the appellate court level. Abe Perlmutter was a 73-year-old man suffering from amyotrophic lateral sclerosis (Lou Gehrig's disease), a fatal disease involving progressive degeneration of muscle and motor ability. At the time of the judicial inquiry, Perlmutter could no longer move, speech was a great strain, and breathing was possible only with the aid of a respirator. The patient was mentally competent and sought removal of the respirator from his trachea. Death would follow the removal within an hour. The judicial opinions don't specify what Perlmutter's life span would have been if the respirator were retained, but the implication was that death could not be forestalled for very long in any event. Describing the patient's condition as a "never ending physical torture," the lower court authorized the removal of the respirator.[2] The highest state court in Florida affirmed the decision on the basis of a terminally ill patient's purported constitutional right to discontinue "extraordinary" treatment.

Most American courts would support the decision reached in *Satz.* Many of the judicial expressions honoring patient choice come in the context of incompetent patients, but this does not diminish their credibility or force. In *Quinlan,* for example, the New Jersey Supreme Court was technically considering only the prerogative of the guardian of the comatose patient. But in doing so, the court observed: "[W]e have no doubt . . . that if Karen were herself miraculously lucid for an interval

. . . and perceptive of her irreversible condition, she could effectively decide upon discontinuance of the life-support apparatus. . . ."[3] The Supreme Court of the State of Washington recently declared in a similar context involving a comatose patient: "[A]n adult who is incurably and terminally ill has a constitutional right of privacy that encompasses the right to refuse treatment that serves only to prolong the dying process. . . ."[4]

Most courts would also endorse the spirit of *Satz*. The Florida court viewed its decision to uphold Mr. Perlmutter's decision to resist further treatment as "an expression of the sanctity of individual free choice and self-determination as fundamental constitutents of life."[5] This language itself was borrowed from a prior Massachusetts opinion[6] and has also been cited approvingly by other state courts. These expressions reflect a current running deep in the American jurisprudence of the last twenty years. That current regards human dignity as embodying individual self-determination in the context of the dying process, at least where choice of medical treatment is an issue.

All courts recognize that there are a variety of claims and interests which might be arrayed against a patient's prerogative to refuse life-preserving medical treatment. The most commonly cited concerns are a state interest in preservation of life, or in promotion of respect for the sanctity of life, and physicians' interests in practicing medicine according to their best professional judgment. A patient's decision to renounce life-preserving measures may pose some tension with these interests. But with regard to a terminal patient facing imminent death, these state interests have not prevailed in the judicial arena and are not likely to prevail.

Sanctity of life is indeed the foundation of a free society, and the state has an indisputable interest in the preservation of life. That legitimate interest is reflected both in the state's general police power (authority to protect public safety), and in a variety of paternalistic legislation (dealing with motorcycle helmets, gambling, drug abuse, and suicide, among other things) aimed in substantial part at safeguarding the individual against himself. In the context of a dying patient refusing medical treatment, strong countervailing interests in bodily integrity and self-determination are confronted. In the balancing process which ensues when a court considers whether a dying patient is entitled to reject further life-preserving treatment, the possible affront to patient choice and autonomy looms large, while the possible harm to the state interest in promoting respect for the sanctity of life seems remote and abstract.

Deference to a terminally ill patient's definition of excessive suffering does not entail a repudiation of society's traditional concern for preserving life and encouraging respect for the sanctity of life. The patient resisting further treatment in this setting is not intent on repudiating life, but on avoiding a prolonged, distasteful dying process. There is no assault on the body or active destruction of life; natural processes are simply allowed to run their course without artificial intervention. Tolerance of the patient's choice to resist treatment reflects concern for individual self-determination, bodily integrity, avoidance of suffering, and empathy with an individual's effort to shape his or her dying process, rather than deprecation of life's value. Judicial acquiescence in a patient's determination is thus impelled by profound respect for individual autonomy, as an integral part of human dignity, and not by any disregard or disdain for the value or sanctity of life.

On occasion, courts will assert that the legitimate government interest in the preservation of life "wanes" as the life span of the patient becomes more and more attenuated and his or her condition deteriorates. This seems to me an ingenuous and wrong suggestion. From a legal perspective, respect for the sanctity of life and for human dignity is not altered by the duration and quality of the remaining existence. For example, state interests in the preservation of innocent life against unsolicited destruction are as strong in the case of an elderly, decrepit person as in the case of a young and vigorous one. What is determinative in the context of a medical patient rejecting life-preserving treatment is the injection of individual interests in self-determination and bodily integrity which have gained considerable respect in American society generally, and in the legal sphere in particular. In other words, the state interest in the sanctity of life does not hinge on the prospective duration or quality of a patient's existence; the state interest is simply overridden by countervailing individual interests. The real test of this thesis comes in the possible extension of the "right" to refuse life-saving medical treatment in the context of a potentially salvageable patient—a topic which is addressed later in this chapter.

Another judicial concern in the context of dying patients refusing life-preserving treatment is the physician's interest in exercising professional judgment without risking civil or criminal liability. Some physicians may be fearful of liability for honoring a patient's request that life-preserving therapy be withheld. The jurisprudence surrounding dying patients is of relatively recent origin, and there may be little judicial precedent in some jurisdictions. In some cases, the legislative prescription of "living wills," for the direction of terminal care, creates confusion about the procedures which must be followed in order for patient choice to be honored. Sometimes, a physician may be fearful of misjudging the patient's competency at the time of making a request for termination of care. Other physicians may be so adamant about prolonging life that they would have scrupled objections to withholding or removing life-preserving measures. For all these reasons, professional flexibility or preference may be cramped if the dying patient is deemed entitled to reject life-preserving medical treatment.

These concerns for the unobstructed exercise of medical judgment have not prevailed in judicial consideration of the prerogatives of a terminally ill patient facing imminent death. This result is not surprising. Unfettered exercise of medical judgment has never been deemed a sacrosanct value. Various laws governing narcotics, experimental drugs, and compulsory medical reporting circumscribe medical practice in ways that are not always pleasing or convenient to physicians. The whole doctrine of informed consent is grounded on the premise that a physician's judgment is subservient to a patient's right to self-determination. While it may be harrowing for a physician to determine whether a patient is voluntarily and competently declining life-preserving treatment, this is simply one of numerous inevitably difficult medical determinations. This is the case, for example, when a patient is certified as mentally ill for purposes of civil commitment or when a patient ostensibly consents to medical procedures which have substantial mortal risks. Furthermore, when an unavoidable death lurks, modern medical practice indicates that any ethical dilemma about honoring a patient's choice to resist life-preserving treatment is considerably diminished.

Over the last twenty years, more and more physicians have acknowledged that "palliative" care (aimed at making the patient comfortable but not prolonging his existence) is an acceptable approach in many terminal cases. In regard to the individual physician who has personal reservations about honoring a dying patient's request to be allowed to die, the solution is not imposition of the physician's preferred course of action on the patient. Rather, the physician can withdraw from the case and the patient can be assisted in finding medical personnel who can, in good conscience, honor the patient's choice of medical strategy. In short, medical interests in pursuing professional skills without threat of liability or obtrusive judicial interference do not dictate overriding requests of competent dying patients to forego further life-preserving medical procedures. The tension between patient choice and medical ethics becomes more acute where the resisting patient is salvageable to a healthful existence—a topic addressed below.

The main issue in *Satz*, and the recent cases addressing terminally ill patients facing imminent death, is not the result, but rather the precise locus of the legal right to resist life-preserving treatment. While the Florida court spoke about a constitutionally grounded "right of privacy" as the source of Mr. Perlmutter's prerogative, other state courts, notably New York,[7] have relied on a common law (judicially crafted) right of a patient to determine what is done to his body. This common law right of bodily integrity flows from the widely accepted notion in criminal law and tort law that a person is master of his or her own body, and that an unconsented invasion constitutes either a battery (impermissible touching) or a trespass (impermissible invasion). Patient autonomy and self-determination are also concepts fitting comfortably within traditional common law doctrine.

Still other state courts have endorsed both sources—constitutional and common law. In terms of the resolution of individual cases, the precise source would not matter. For, as will be explained, the contours of the constitutional and common law rights are quite similar. But the locus of the right is important for purposes of ensuring its durability. If the source is the Constitution, the patient's right cannot be altered by legislative tampering, and is less subject to judicial manipulation. Further, source of the right would have implications for the handling of incompetent patients, a subject which will be considered in chapter 3.

The hypothesis that the federal Constitutional right to privacy extends to a competent, terminally ill patient's rejection of life-preserving medical treatment is likely to prevail. While the United States Supreme Court has never resolved the case of a dying medical patient, signposts indicate that it will eventually endorse the position articulated by the *Satz* court, among others. The Supreme Court has previously established that certain aspects of "liberty" are fundamental and entitled to particularly strong protection under the due process clauses of the Fifth and Fourteenth Amendments. While these fundamental aspects of liberty have not been exhaustively defined, existing precedents include within fundamental privacy the notion of bodily integrity, i.e., security from government ordered physical invasions, as well as autonomy or freedom of choice concerning certain intimate personal matters. A woman's decision whether to bear a child is probably the best known example of an aspect of autonomy elevated to the status of fundamental privacy. A dying patient's rejection of life-preserving medical treatment inevitably involves both physical integrity and autonomy concerning an intimate and important matter—dying and the dying process. Consideration of these elements supports the contention that the emerging judicial trend to treat rejection of life-preserving care as a fundamental aspect of liberty will eventually be accepted by the Supreme Court.

Of course, not every intimate or personal matter is covered by the fundamental right to privacy. Such important matters as choice of school companions (private schools) or choice of a living arrangement with several persons have been excluded from the category of fundamental aspects of liberty.[8] Nonetheless, the Supreme Court purports to draw its guidance for defining fundamental privacy from "the traditions and collective conscience of the people."[9] Using this as the guide, evolving societal values and practices point strongly toward the acceptance of a terminally ill patient's prerogative to reject life-preserving medical treatment. Support for this proposition comes from several different indicators of evolving societal values.

State judicial decisions such as that in *Satz* will provide one important index of social values to guide the Supreme Court. In that vein, one court has commented:

> The decision by the incurably ill to forego medical treatment and allow the natural processes of death to follow their inevitable course is so manifestly a 'fundamental' decision in their lives, that it is virtually inconceivable that the right of privacy would *not* apply to it.[10]

This optimistic projection by a lower court judge is by no means determinative. But there are further indices pointing toward recognition that fundamental personal privacy encompasses a dying patient's right to decline life-preserving treatment.

The widespread adoption of "natural death" acts by state legislatures offers an important insight into public attitudes toward the dying medical patient. These statutes, adopted in approximately 35 states, are intended to provide an officially sanctioned avenue for people to determine beforehand their own fate in the event that they are later incompetent when they reach a terminal state. The object is that the patient provide prior binding instructions that certain medical procedures be omitted in the event that an extreme state of debilitation is reached with no hope of recovery.

These "natural death" or "living will" statutes are valuable more for their symbolic than their instrumental value. Their practical utility is limited by overly restrictive preconditions to validity, vague instructions to guide the medical practitioner, and the fact that most people are simply not oriented toward using such documents to address their own dying process. Evolving judicial doctrine seems to provide a more flexible guide for recognizing the prerogatives of competent patients facing death. Nonetheless, the legislative expressions in these statutes offer an important index of the societal importance attached to self-determination in the dying process—an index which will help convince courts that rejection of life-preserving medical care is indeed a fundamental aspect of personal privacy.

The California Natural Death Act[11] provides an illustration. The legislative "findings" there first acknowledge that medical prolongation of the dying process of some terminally ill patients may cause unnecessary pain, suffering and loss of dignity. The legislation also declares that adults possess "the fundamental right to control the decisions relating to . . . their own medical care, including the decision to have life-sustaining procedures withheld or withdrawn in instances of a terminal condition."[12] These expressions, typical of those legislatures which have adopted such natural death acts, bear witness to societal acceptance of individual autonomy to resist prolongation of the dying process.

The traditional common law concern with bodily integrity furnishes another source demonstrating the fundamentality of patient self-determination. Indeed, as has occurred in New York, common law doctrine can serve as an independent legal basis (without reliance on the Constitution) for a terminally ill patient's prerogative to resist life-preserving medical intervention. As early as 1891, the U.S. Supreme Court declared:

> No right is held more sacred, or is more carefully guarded, by the common law, than the right of every individual to the possession and control of his own person, free from all restraint or interference by others, unless by clear and unquestionable authority of law.[13]

More recently, the medical patient's right to bodily control has been embodied in the tort doctrine of informed consent. Under this doctrine, no medical procedure may be performed without a patient's consent, obtained after explanation of the nature of the treatment, substantial risks, and alternative therapies. The doctrine recognizes that the consequence of a physician's explanation and consultation may be a patient's refusal of treatment and assumption of a risk of harm. As expressed by one state court:

> Anglo American law starts with the premise of thorough-going self determination. It follows that each man is considered to be master of his own body, and he may, if he be of sound mind, expressly prohibit the performance of life-saving surgery, or other medical treatment. A doctor might well believe that an operation or form of treatment is desirable or necessary, but the law does not permit him to substitute his own judgment for that of the patient by any form of artifice or deception.[14]

These principles have won widespread recognition not just in judicial and legislative circles, but in medical circles as well. The recent reports of the President's Commission for the Study of Ethical Problems in Medicine and Biomedical and Behavioral Research (hereinafter cited as the "President's Commission") place careful emphasis on patient self-determination, even in the context of life and death decisions. Those reports accepted self-determination as the key not only to defining what is really "good" for each patient, but also as an element of human worth and autonomy that deserves respect. One Commission report cites respect for patient decision-making as "one of the wellsprings of a democracy."[15] This claim might be exaggerated as applied to all democracies, but it accurately conveys the high value traditionally placed by American society on self-determination. Even in the context of the cherished societal interest in preserving human life, respect for autonomy has frequently prevailed. This has sometimes involved societal acquiescence in decision-making which might be deemed imprudent or irrational from a "logical" perspective. Deference to individual decisions to smoke or drink alcohol offers one example. Deference to a mental patient's refusal of anti-psychotic medication, even if such medicine would utlimately benefit the patient, offers another illustration.[16] Even an accused criminal, under the rubric of exercising a constitutional right to counsel, can choose the imprudent course of conducting his own defense—all in the interest of "dignity and autonomy."[17]

In short, it's not at all surprising that individual self-determination has been widely deemed to embody a terminally ill patient's prerogative to reject life-preserving medical care in the context of intolerable suffering and imminent death. Acceptance of the prerogative by state judicial, legislative, and medical sources augers well for its eventual enshrinement by the U.S. Supreme Court as a matter of an emerging constitutional right of privacy.

Even without reliance on the federal Constitution, the common law doctrine of informed consent provides a firm basis for legal recognition of the competent, terminally ill patient's prerogative to resist life-preserving medical care. That doctrine entitles the patient, not only to be informed about the shape and course of prospective medical treatment, but to withhold consent where the prospective medical intervention is personally distasteful. The common law right is grounded on the same notions of autonomy and self-determination that lie at the core of the asserted constitutional privacy right.

Indeed, there appears to be a judicial trend to rely more on the common law prerogative and less on constitutional bases in discussions of a "right" to resist life-preserving treatment. In an important 1985 decision called *In re Conroy*,[18] the New Jersey Supreme Court—the same body which in its 1976 *Quinlan* decision gave great impetus to the notion of a constitutional right to resist life-preserving care—grounded its discussion of a competent patient's status on a person's common law right to determine when, and if, to accept medical intervention. Other courts seem to be moving in the same direction.[19]

The reason for this recent trend is probably that the Supreme Court has shown some signs of narrowing its concept of fundamental privacy, confining it primarily to personal choices surrounding reproduction, marriage, and family life.[20] By establishing common law informed consent as an alternative rationale for honoring a patient's prerogative to resist life-preserving treatment, the courts assure the upholding of the patient's prerogative regardless of the vicissitudes of constitutional interpretation. (The prerogative is then secure so long as legislatures are willing to accept the judicially evolved doctrine).

In terms of content of the patient's prerogative, locating the right in common law doctrine rather than the federal Constitution will not have major ramifications. All courts which have accepted the right of privacy in the dying patient context have regarded the constitutional right as congruent with the common law right. As noted above, anchoring the patient's prerogative in constitutional doctrine would help preserve it against legislative alteration. Yet anchoring the prerogative in the tort doctrine of informed consent may actually have its own advantages. First, the patient does not have to worry about "state action" (government involvement) in order to assert his right. His legal claim to determine his medical course is as applicable to a private hospital or private practitioner as it is to a government-sponsored institution subject to the Fifth or Fourteenth Amendments. Further, the opportunity may be enhanced for collecting damages when medical sources override the patient's right to refuse treatment. The patient, or patient's estate, can invoke the well-established tort doctrine of informed consent without having to cope with the more uncertain strictures of constitutional torts. Through this common law claim, the moribund patient is likely to have a firmer legal footing in his effort to compel medical sources to respect his determinations in shaping the dying process.

The reality is that the threat of damage claims is not an imposing one in the context of a terminally ill patient facing imminent death. Though there is a potential claim for unnecessarily prolonged suffering,[21] a court or jury may be sympathetic with the physician's plaint that he was seeking to preserve life, or that he was uncertain about the patient's competence to make a life-rejecting decision. Nonetheless, any significant threat of a lawsuit—with all its burdens and inconveniences—may have an impact on ongoing medical practice. Advocates of patient's prerogatives can therefore welcome the two arrows—constitutional privacy and informed consent—now in the legal quiver of the dying patient seeking to reject life-preserving medical treatment. A further question is whether the rights of self-determination and bodily integrity will be extended to include patient rejection of life-preserving medical treatment in situations where death is not both imminent and unavoidable.

Patients Facing Unavoidable but Non-Imminent Death

Virtually all "natural death" or "living will" statutes dictate that the patient's death be "imminent" before a statutory obligation arises to honor the now incompetent patient's prior instruction to terminate life-preserving medical machinery. Moreover, medical institutions and physicians are oriented toward extending life whenever possible. A patient's request to have life-sustaining care withdrawn despite the fact that a moribund existence is preservable for a considerable period therefore runs counter to the normal institutional inclinations. Consequently, institutions tend to contest or resist efforts by a patient to terminate care when death is not imminent (for the sake of discussion, I'll use survival for a week or more as the period defining nonimminence).

A poignant reminder of this tendency came in late 1984, when a California hospital resisted the plea of William Bartling, a 70-year-old man suffering from five potentially fatal conditions—cancer, emphysema, chronic respiratory failure, arteriosclerosis, and an abdominal aneurysm. The patient had requested to be removed from a life-sustaining ventilator. The hospital's explanation for disregarding the patient's choice was, in part, that death was not sufficiently imminent. Despite some medical projections that the patient would last another year, he died within weeks, still attached to the despised respirator. The hospital inherited a lawsuit contending that the dying patient's rights had been violated.

Despite the institutional hesitation to recognize a patient's choice of death, as reflected in the recent California incident, the cases tend to endorse the prerogative of a terminally ill, competent patient to resist life-sustaining treatment even if a moribund existence is preservable for a considerable period—at least so long as the prospective existence is a dismal one. In the California case regarding Mr. Bartling, for example, a state appellate court confirmed (months after the patient died while still on the ventilator) that the patient's request to have life-support equipment disconnected should have been respected.[22] The decision was based on the right of a competent adult to refuse medical treatment, a right derived by the court both from common law and constitutional (right of privacy) sources.

A 1982 New York case, *Lydia E. Hall Hospital,*[23] provides another illustration. There, the patient, forty-one-year-old Peter Cinque, had suffered from diabetes since childhood. By October 1982 the diabetes had produced a number of seriously debilitating conditions. Cinque was then suffering from final stage kidney disease, blindness, effects of a double amputation, gastro-intestinal bleeding, a bleeding ulcer, and calcification of the aorta. He was undergoing kidney dialysis three times each week, four hours each session, for a total of twelve hours per week. His life expectancy with continued dialysis was six months; without it, he would die within one week. In October 1982, Cinque carefully explained to his family and physicians his decision to forego further dialysis treatment. He had concluded that his debilitated status and continuous suffering associated with the burdensome treatment warranted a termination of the life-prolonging treatment. Cinque's family supported his decision, but the hospital resisted and obtained a temporary court order maintaining dialysis pending a final judicial determination.

By the time the final judicial decision was rendered, Cinque had become comatose and hence incompetent. The court treated the case as one involving a termination decision sought by a competent patient, considering Cinque's state at the moment he first sought to have dialysis ended. The court ruled that Cinque's decision to forego dialysis must be respected. Citing the "constant and severe pain" caused by Cinque's various afflictions, and referring to the patient's "irreversible and terminal" condition, the court found that Cinque was entitled to escape prolongation of his personally distasteful status.[24] No particular reference was made to the fact that his existence was preservable for another six months. In early 1984, newspapers reported a similar ruling in a New York case involving an 85-year-old former college president suffering from the effects of a prior stroke, high fever, and infection. Rejecting a nursing home's petition for judicial intervention, the judge allowed the patient to continue resisting intravenous feeding and to starve to death.[25]

The New Jersey Supreme Court's *Conroy* decision,[26] in January 1985, will further dispel any notion that life-preserving treatment can be resisted only when death is imminent. There, the court endorsed possible termination of life-preserving treatment for patients whose life expectancy is one year or less. (The case primarily dealt with the handling of incompetent patients, but the court's position on imminence of death applies a fortiori to competent patients).

The *Conroy* opinion effectively recognizes that the various interests at stake in the effort of a terminally ill patient to resist medical intervention do not hinge on the "imminence" of the moment of death. The bodily integrity which is at stake in a patient's refusal of treatment is as applicable six months before the potential moment of death as six minutes before. The patient's autonomy or self-determination interest does not materialize only when the dying process has reached a stage when death is imminent. The autonomy interest is in shaping the dying process—that is, in determining for oneself when the burdens of the preservable existence outweigh the prospective benefits of medical intervention. "Death with dignity" can include avoidance of months (or years) of suffering which sometime accompany the dying process.

The uncertainty of medical prediction about the precise moment of death also dictates that the patient's prerogative not be confined to situations where death is certified as "imminent." Otherwise, many patients will end up suffering an excruciating death—maintained on machinery against the patient's will up to the last moment—because of a physician's honest but erroneous projection that death is not yet imminent. This is precisely what occurred in the *Bartling* case mentioned earlier.

Cases like *Conroy, Lydia E. Hall Hospital,* and *Bartling,* in effect recognize a corollary of the competent, terminally ill patient's prerogative to resist life-preserving medical treatment—a prerogative to determine when the prospective moribund existence is so dismal and distasteful that further resistance to the inevitable dying process can be foregone. The judgment being made is, that while death may not be imminent, if medical intervention is maintained, the remaining existence is so burdensome that from the perspective of the patient death is preferable to continued treatment. This is a quality of life judgment. It involves an assessment of both physical and emotional pain. It is both a legitimate and an inevitable exercise in the context of death and dying and decisions to withhold or withdraw life-preserving medical care.

The status of many terminally ill cancer patients offers an example. Chemotherapy may offer a probability of a "remission" for months or more. But the period may be accompanied by hair loss, noxious side effects of the drugs, emaciation, and emotional pain connected to feelings of dependency or loss of self-respect. Each patient will have to determine his or her own tolerances and priorities. In an era in which patient self-determination is exalted, it is simply inconceivable that the terminally ill cancer patient's choice to forego chemotherapy would not be honored. This is so even if the patient's decision means hastening a death which would be non-imminent if medical intervention were accepted. In effect, the patient is being permitted to define the "pain" of the remaining existence—in terms of not only physical discomfort, but of dependency, embarrassment, isolation, or other emotional burdens. (The same phenomenon is present when patients are permitted to forego life-preserving care even though they would be salvageable to a normal life span—for example, when a gangrene patient is allowed to resist a life-preserving amputation. This topic will be addressed in the next subsection.)

The irrelevance of imminence of death is brought home starkly in the context of degenerative nervous system diseases such as Alzheimer's disease or Huntington's chorea. The latter is an irreversible neurological disorder whose symptoms include uncontrollable twitching and contortion of the face and hands, as well as progressive dementia, i.e., deterioration of intellectual function. If a particular patient, while still competent, fixes a point beyond which resistance is too torturous—either because of present strains or prospective deterioration—that patient ought to be able to dictate cessation of life-preserving medical interventions. The contrary position, under which the patient can seek relief only when death is "imminent," violates the patient's autonomy to define when the prospective moribund period is too burdensome or dismal to bear.

The "imminence" issue arises in an interesting context when a patient with a long-term fatal illness is stricken with a potentially fatal but curable second illness. As examples, one can imagine an AIDS or Huntington's chorea victim who is stricken with pneumonia long before the moment when the underlying disease would be fatal. Can the competent patient reject treatment for the pneumonia as a means of avoiding the prospective suffering which would eventually accompany the underlying fatal condition? Even before the degenerative illness has reached its most debilitating stages? Judicial precedent on the issue is sparse. But I have no trouble concluding that the patient *should* be allowed to reject treatment to avoid prospective suffering just as he or she would be allowed to resist treatment for the underlying fatal condition. There could be little dispute about this if the underlying condition were already painful and debilitating. I doubt that the prospect of a period of grace before the final stages of the fatal condition ought to change the result. Part of the principle of self-determination and autonomy at stake here is the prerogative to define for oneself what is painful and torturous, both physically and psychologically. The anxiety prompted by the prospective deterioration and incapacity may constitute a real form of suffering to the hypothetical terminally ill patient.

By choosing to succumb to an intervening illness, without allowing the underlying illness to run its full course, the patient does sacrifice a grace period during which some miraculous cure might materialize. Still, this is simply another factor for consideration in the patient's informed decision about whether to undertake life-preserving therapy. A prerogative to refuse treatment includes a prerogative to renounce any potential miraculous cure.

In practice, physicians certainly collaborate at times with competent patients (and with families of incompetent patients) to refrain from treating a terminally ill patient's new, intervening pathology. For example, the deteriorating patient and physician may agree to a "do not resuscitate" (DNR) order in the patient's chart. The understanding is that cardiac arrest will not be treated if and when it occurs. Some physicians also acknowledge that fever or infection will not be treated—with the consequence that the patient may die—in some instances of severely deteriorated patients.[27] Thus, the concept is accepted among some practitioners that a terminally ill patient may choose not to resist an intervening illness even though the patient's death may be significantly accelerated.

A further question is whether the competent patient's prerogative to define his own "suffering"—including subjective emotional concerns—allows the patient to use altruistic factors, such as avoidance of economic and emotional burdens to survivors, in choosing to reject life-preserving treatment. The answer is almost certainly yes. For some terminally ill patients engaged in assessing when life has become excessively burdensome, it is quite natural to be anxious about the various strains facing close relatives. And it is natural to include such considerations in determining which course of treatment or nontreatment to pursue. Courts have sometimes noted that emotional and financial relief to survivors is at least one of the "ancillary benefits" flowing from a decision to terminate life-preserving care. And the recent President's Commission, in its report entitled "Deciding to Forego Life-Sustaining Treatment," noted the appropriateness of considering economic costs in the context of the terminally ill patient.[28] Thus, altruistic concerns can be a legitimate element in the calculus of the terminally ill patient deciding when existence has become intolerably painful or burdensome.

This discussion of a terminal patient's prerogative to define the "pain" of a remaining existence, and to dictate an end to medical intervention even when death is nonimminent, is suffused with "quality of life" assessments by the patient. The quality of remaining existence is inevitably a principal criterion in the competent patient's decision whether to initiate life-preserving machinery, and whether to withdraw it once initiated.

Such quality of life considerations are certainly not foreign to physicians handling terminally ill patients. Much of the medical writing of the sixties and seventies agonizing over how to handle such patients is suffused with concern about how to identify those patients whose remaining existence is so devoid of "meaningful" function that life-preserving measures may be omitted. Polls of surgeons indicate that their attitude about life-saving brain surgery changes radically if there is a significant chance that the patient will survive with impaired mental functioning. A far lower percentage is in favor of operating in the latter event.

On the other hand, there are physicians who will be troubled by a patient's own negative assessment of the quality of remaining existence and about the patient's determination to reject life-preserving treatment. Those physicians are entitled to preserve their integrity by refusing to implement a course which they consider unconscionable. But they cannot impose their personal judgment on the patient. Their proper course is to withdraw from the case, and to facilitate the patient's obtaining another practitioner who is willing to follow the patient's chosen course. The same principle is applicable where dying patients who are potentially salvageable to a "normal" life span resist medical intervention.

Patients with Fatal Conditions Whose Lives Are Salvageable

While some sources speak—erroneously, I think—of imminence of death as a prerequisite to a competent patient's right to reject life-preserving treatment, many more state a precondition that the patient's condition be terminal, i.e., that the dying process be irreversible before a patient's "right" arises. For example, many of the previously described "natural death acts" require that a patient's condition be terminal before a physician or hospital is obligated to honor a "living will." And courts which have found a constitutional basis for a patient's prerogative to resist life-preserving treatment commonly include, in defining the bounds of the constitutional privacy right, the notion that approaching death be unavoidable. Their premise appears to be that government's legitimate interest in the preservation and sanctity of human life is overridden only where the patient is not renouncing a salvageable existence, but rather is simply ceasing to resist an inexorable dying process.

The frequent reference to unremediable terminal illness is readily understandable in this emerging and relatively fledgling area of law. In hesitatingly mapping out the contours of a patient's prerogative to resist life-preserving treatment, the courts have most readily grasped concepts consistent with preexisting legal doctrine and with evolving medical practice. First, the courts had to fit their analysis of the handling of dying medical patients to existing legal strictures surrounding homicide, suicide, and torts. As will be shown in detail in chapter 2, those strictures were most elastic where the patient's choice entailed allowing an inexorable dying process to continue—letting nature take its course. This accounts for the frequent reference in relevant judicial opinions to the notion that medical intervention was merely postponing the inevitable moment of death.

Further, the courts naturally sought guidance in this area from emerging mores of medical practice. And the clearest medical concensus to emerge has been that some patients ought to be able to refuse life-preserving treatment in the context of a nonreversible disease process. The medical community relatively early recognized that, for some dying medical patients, palliative care and comfort were more appropriate than active life-sustaining intervention. Along these lines, the recent President's Commission endorsed refusals of treatment by patients "dying of a disease process that cannot be arrested."[29] Such medical positions have inevitably influenced judicial development of doctrine in this area.

Some courts have ventured forth and have upheld a patient's prerogative to resist life-preserving therapy even where that therapy could have restored the patient to a "healthy" condition—i.e., where the patient's condition was not really terminal. In such instances, there is a strong tension between self-determination as expressed in patient choice and preferred medical practice. Physicians, given their choice, would intervene and seek to salvage such patients. Hospitals will commonly oppose such patients' choice to resist treatment and will seek judicial guidance.

Where the resisting patient is salvageable to a healthful existence, the medical personnel (and judges when their intervention is sought) are faced with an anguishing dilemma. By respecting patient choice, they are allowing a "needless" death to occur. This runs counter both to professional judgment and normal legal prescripts. The situation is particularly wrenching when the patient does not really wish to die, but is only abiding by religious dictates. Religious freedom, bodily integrity, or individual self-determination may appear to be evanescent or ephemeral principles in the face of an immediate threat to life.

A recent trial court decision in New York, *Randolph v. City of New York*,[30] illustrates both the medical dilemma and the judicial empathy evoked. The patient was a forty-five-year-old woman, mother of three children, who had been admitted to the hospital to undergo a caesarian section (at the birth of her fourth child) and a tubal ligation. The patient had been explicitly warned about a hazard of hemorrhage, but as a devout Jehovah's witness the patient had made it clear that she wanted no blood transfusion, even in the face of death. The attending physician had agreed in principle to respect the patient's religious scruples. He adhered to his agreement even after complications arose following the birth of a healthy infant at 11:45 A.M. In response to hemorrhage the physician at noon administered a non-blood fluid to the circulatory system in order to compensate in some fashion for fluid loss. By 12:30 P.M. the patient had lost 3,000 cc's of blood, half her normal volume, and was in critical condition. At 12:45 P.M. the attending physician, having thought about the patient's children (including her one-hour-old infant), began to transfuse one unit (500 cc's) of blood. At 1:30 P.M. a second transfusion of one unit was administered. At 2:00 P.M. the patient was pronounced dead. A law suit ensued in which the patient's heirs sought to hold the physician and hospital liable. A jury awarded $2.5 million, a figure which was reduced by the trial court to $1 million.

The trial judge, Justice Bambrick, expressed empathy for the attending physician's plight—torn between a desire to honor the patient's wish (including fear of liability for overriding the patient's choice) and an urge to perform the lifesaving processes that medical practice would normally dictate. The judge saw the physician as drifting on a "professional life raft in between a legal Scylla and Charybdis." Justice Bambrick also saw the physician's legal course in the difficult circumstances as chartable. According to Justice Bambrick's opinion upholding the physician's liability, the doctor could not have been faulted if he had simply withheld transfusions based on the patient's request not to receive blood. New York tort law regards the patient's right to make an informed direction of treatment as paramount vis a vis a doctor's preference to provide life-saving care. Overriding the wishes of a competent adult patient would constitute an actionable tort.

Yet the physician's liability in *Randolph* was not grounded on the overriding of the patient's will. (Certainly, the patient's monetary damages from the decision to transfuse were nowhere near $1 million; if the physician had followed the patient's directions the patient would simply have died an hour earlier). The big damage award flowed from negligent administration of the transfusions. Once the physician decided to override the patient's directions, the patient could have been saved if the transfusions had been administered at a proper rate. In short, the doctor's decision to try and save the patient proved so costly not because of the injury to the patient's autonomy interest, but because of the negligent course of medical intervention.

There are, and will be for some time, divergent judicial approaches to the competent patient who rejects life-saving medical treatment even though the patient's condition is not necessarily fatal. Some courts will probably balk at authorizing termination of life-preserving care of a salvageable patient. There are hints from both *Quinlan* and *Saikewicz,* two of the leading decisions in the death and dying area, along these lines. Justice Liacos of the Massachusetts Supreme Judicial Court, the author of the *Saikewicz* opinion, has contended that the Massachusetts court was only endorsing the prerogative of a dying patient to act "reasonably and rationally."[31] Many instances when a nonterminal patient rejects life-preserving care might be labeled "irrational," allowing medical intervention under the Liacos formula.

The New Jersey Supreme Court in *Quinlan* hinted that its endorsement of termination decisions might be confined to situations where death was inevitable and the prospective interim existence dismal. That court sought to distinguish its own prior decision which had mandated treatment for a twenty-two-year-old accident victim who had resisted a life-saving blood transfusion.[32] In the prior case, the patient had been "salvable to long life and vibrant health" while Karen Ann Quinlan faced a permanently comatose state.[33] A possible implication there was that the New Jersey court was confining the patient's "right" to resist life-preserving intervention to situations where death or its equivalent, permanent coma, is medically unavoidable.

As noted, judicial reluctance to allow salvageable patients to resist life-saving treatment is grounded both on sympathy with medical interests involved and on concern for the state interest in the preservation of life. For reasons that will be detailed in chapter 2, a refusal of life-saving medical treatment is not synonymous with "suicide." Nonetheless, state efforts to curb suicide through detention of persons making attempts at suicide and threatened punishment of anyone "aiding or abetting" a suicide confirm that preservation of life is generally deemed a legitimate and strong governmental interest. There is some temptation for the courts to say, as did one respected jurist: "if the state may interrupt one mode of self-destruction [suicide], it may with equal authority interfere with the other [refusal of life-saving medical treatment]."[34]

I respectfully suggest that judicial doctrine ought to evolve and is evolving in a different direction—toward respecting patient choice to resist life-preserving treatment even where the patient is salvageable to what most observers would regard as a desirable level of existence. The thesis is that patient self-determination or autonomy is an essential part of the human dignity cherished by American society. That dignity is impinged when a competent person's voluntary choice is overridden, even where the patient's determination is distasteful to the medical and judicial personnel confronting the situation. Perhaps the offense to human dignity and autonomy exists in its most objectionable form where treatment is forced on a dying patient who is intent on maintaining dignity in the face of an irremediable dying process. But an offense exists as well when the will of a salvageable patient is overridden.

Some courts would eliminate the patient's prerogative to resist life-preserving treatment in situations where the patient is salvageable to "a relatively normal, healthy life."[35] In effect, such a court sustains the patient's ordering of values—sacrifice of life in favor of religious scruples or in avoidance of a subjectively painful existence—only when the court feels that the potential existence in issue is not really worth preserving. This is not a very seemly judicial posture. That realization recently prompted the New Jersey Supreme Court, in its *Conroy* decision, to renounce (in dictum) any distinction between the self-determination prerogatives of a salvageable patient and an irreversibly moribund patient. The court observed:

> [A] young, generally healthy person, if competent, has the same right to decline life-saving medical treatment as a competent elderly person who is terminally ill. Of course, a patient's decision to accept or reject medical treatment may be influenced by his medical condition, treatment, and prognosis; nevertheless, a competent person's common-law and constitutional rights do not depend on the quality or value of his life.[36]

There are two significant strands of judicial authority consistent with this emerging thesis that the patient's prerogative to resist life-saving treatment extends to a patient salvageable to a normal life span. One set of cases acquiesces in patient decisions where the life which would be preserved is disabled and therefore distasteful to the patient. A second line of authority (including the *Randolph* case in New York dealing with blood transfusions) acquiesces in patient decisions motivated by religious principles.

The first group is typified by *Lane v. Candura*,[37] a 1978 decision by a lower court in Massachusetts. There, the court upheld the decision by a seventy-seven-year-old widow suffering from gangrene of the leg to resist a life-saving amputation. The widow didn't wish to live as an invalid or in a nursing home, she didn't wish to burden her children, she had no confidence in the outcome of the operation, and she had been generally unhappy since her husband had died. The court ruled that the patient had a right to reject treatment, even if the decision might be deemed irrational or unwise by many people's standards. The decision was grounded on constitutional privacy and self-determination. In effect, the court was allowing the patient to dictate her own treatment according to her personal values and preferences. To her, the specter of a disabled existence as an aged amputee was more distasteful than the prospective death from the gangrene rotting her leg. This personal ordering of tastes and priorities is at the core of patient self-determination.

A similar result was obtained in a 1978 lower court decision in New Jersey in which a seventy-two-year-old recluse was allowed to reject an amputation needed to arrest gangrene.[38] The patient's decision meant death within three weeks. But the court would not intervene even though the patient did not wish to die and hoped for a miracle. In both of these refusal of amputation cases, the judges apparently had some empathy with the value judgment reflected in the patients' determination to avoid a prospective handicapped existence. A similar judicial attitude has been displayed in a few cases expressing willingness to allow kidney dialysis patients to forego the burdensome process of being connected to a dialysis machine up to twelve hours per week—even though the rejection of dialysis meant death.[39] Judges can empathize with the considerable demands placed on the dialysis patient from a physical, emotional, and financial perspective, and hence can understand a patient's plea to be relieved from the strains.

There is some temptation to regard the dialysis or amputation cases[40] as a special breed because of the considerable bodily invasion involved. Indeed, the courts in such cases do make reference to a patient's interest in bodily integrity and to the magnitude of the prospective bodily invasion entailed in an amputation (or in physical linkage to a dialysis machine). The *Quinlan* court in its groundbreaking decision had also contended that a patient's right to privacy increases as the degree of bodily invasion grows.[41] Nonetheless, these cases are better viewed as self-determination or autonomy decisions in which the gross bodily invasion merely offers an incidental or makeweight argument for nonintervention. There are many other decisions recognizing patient autonomy to resist treatment where the bodily invasions are fairly minimal. These include instances when the prospective treatment was merely a blood transfusion, or oral administration of medicine, or even maintenance of intravenous feeding, as in the 1984 New York case involving an eighty-five-year-old former college president who was permitted to starve himself to death.[42]

I suggest that the key to all these decisions is self-determination—freedom to implement personal value choices and, in particular, to define when a prospective existence is too burdensome or torturous to warrant resistance to a potentially fatal medical condition. I doubt that the gangrene patient resisting amputation is bothered more by the prospective bodily invasion through surgery than by the rotting flesh which he is choosing to endure. What is distasteful to these patients is the prospective incapacity and dependency after the amputation. The lesson of the amputation cases ought to be that patient autonomy includes the prerogative to resist life-preserving treatment where the existence to be preserved would represent a subjective hell for the patient.

A separate line of cases has upheld patient autonomy to resist life-preserving treatment—even though the patient was salvageable to a physically healthful existence—where religious scruples motivated the patient's determination. Most of these cases involve Jehovah's Witnesses, a religious group which believes that blood transfusions violate biblical injunctions. Many adherents of this sect consider a blood transfusion to be a serious religious transgression and would rather die than receive one.

Perhaps the most articulate statement for the position opposing interference in a patient's religiously motivated rejection of life-preserving treatment is found in a 1965 Illinois case, *In re Brooks' Estate*.[43] There, the patient, a female Jehovah's Witness, refused a transfusion necessary to the treatment of a peptic ulcer. The patient had a spouse and adult children, but they did not oppose her refusal. In a unanimous decision, the Supreme Court of Illinois upheld the patient's right to determine her own fate. Although a hospital representative asserted an overriding societal interest in protecting human life, the court perceived no threat to the public health, safety, or welfare sufficient to outweigh the patient's interest in religious freedom. The court commented:

> Even though we may consider [Mrs. Brooks'] beliefs unwise, foolish or ridiculous, in the absence of an overriding danger to society we may not permit interference therewith . . . for the sole purpose of compelling her to accept medical treatment forbidden by her religious principles, and previously refused by her with full knowledge of the probable consequences.[44]

In a 1972 case, *In re Osborne*,[45] the patient was a thirty-four-year-old Jehovah's Witness suffering from internal bleeding and rejecting a critical blood transfusion. The court denied the hospital's application for a court order overriding the patient's determination. The patient's interest in religious freedom and autonomy was deemed to prevail over the societal interest in preserving life and promoting the sanctity of life.

The cases concerning religiously motivated refusals of life-preserving treatment are not unanimous. But, by and large, the cases where patient choice was not fully respected involve special circumstances. Either the patient's competency was seriously in question, or the patient's religious scruples were such that they were not really contravened when the court ordered a transfusion (as opposed to the patient's *consenting* to a transfusion).[46]

In a few instances, courts have used the presence of minor children (who might be harmed by the demise of their parent resisting a blood transfusion) to justify judicial mandating of treatment.[47] By keeping the parent alive, the child presumably benefits emotionally, via continued love and reassurance from the parent, and economically, by continued financial support. However, while a state may indeed have legitimate interests in the emotional and economic well-being of these prospective survivors, these interests would not usually justify interference with a patient's decision to resist a blood transfusion.

Parental conduct which causes serious emotional harm to offspring is concededly a compelling basis for state intervention, as illustrated in the child neglect laws found in every American jurisdiction. But the loss of a parent will not always cause serious emotional harm, especially if the remaining spouse or family can provide a loving environment. Moreover, a parent is allowed to separate from a household, divorce, move away, or even surrender a child for adoption despite potential infliction of emotional wounds. Such unintended inflictions of emotional harm do not generally lead to state intervention. Judicial intervention in such instances would provoke indignant outcries about state interference with personal liberty. It is arguable, then, that the loss of one of two parents because of a parent's adherence to religious or personal convictions in declining treatment—while relevant to the state's interest in a child's emotional well-being—is an inadequate basis for judicial intervention. I suspect that the emotional well-being of surviving children is not really what's motivating judicial intervention in the rare instances when a parent's rejection of life-saving treatment is overridden. Rather, these courts are simply uncomfortable with the "illogic" of the patient's decision to resist life-saving care.

A state also has a legitimate interest in ensuring that children are not left without economic support. There is a selfish interest in avoiding new burdens to the public welfare rolls, and a paternalistic interest in safeguarding the economic conditions of a child. Moreover, avoidance of state economic burdens has, in some instances, served as a justification for state conduct which would otherwise be considered to impermissibly impinge on personal liberty. Motorcycle helmet laws—sustained in some jurisdictions against constitutional challenges—provide one example. Yet concern for the economic interests of survivors would not warrant a flat judicial refusal to tolerate a parent's resistance to a life-saving blood transfusion.

The economic factors justifying judicial intervention are not present in every case of a parent's refusal of treatment. A court should at least inquire whether, even if a parent dies, the economic well-being of survivors will be safeguarded. This was the approach taken by several courts which acquiesced in a parent's rejection of a life-saving transfusion when the court was assured that the children's economic future was secure.[48] In the recent New York trial court decision described above (the *Randolph* case involving a female Jehovah's Witness who was mother to four children), the court ruled that the state's interest in protection of minors was not compelling if a parent remains who is capable of supporting the children.

The whole notion that a patient's religiously grounded refusal of treatment might be overridden because the patient is not affluent enough to assure that dependents will never be wards of the state is suspect. It is true that the state is not usually constitutionally obligated to subsidize the exercise of legal rights by poor persons. This was established in the abortion funding cases. Nonetheless, hinging judicial respect for an adult's decision about life-preserving treatment on the family's financial circumstances may ultimately prove unpalatable to the judiciary. The practical effect is to tell the patient that his or her convictions will not be respected because the family does not have enough money. This is an unsavory result, especially considering the overall magnitude of the government fiscal interest involved. A rather small number of people can be expected to spurn life-saving medical treatment when they know their family will be left impecunious. Again I suggest that the few courts which raise this economic rationale for judicial intervention are masking their personal distaste for the patient's particular choice. The only convincing rationale for overriding a religiously grounded rejection of a blood transfusion is where the patient indicates that a state ordered intervention (as opposed to the patient's voluntarily submitting to a transfusion) would not really constitute a significant affront to the patient's scruples.[49]

The bulk of judicial precedent upholds the religiously motivated patient's right to reject a life-saving blood transfusion. In this line of cases, as in the amputation cases, self-determination and autonomy are found to prevail even in the face of government's legitimate interest in promoting respect for the sanctity of life. Nor can the right involved be confined to religiously grounded refusals of treatment. Normally, religious scruples are not regarded as any more sacrosanct against government interference than other philosophical or conscientious scruples. Thus, a dying patient who has a philosophical antipathy to blood transfusions has as much right to resist a life-saving transfusion as a Jehovah's Witness. Even without a religious prop to a patient's decision, and even without a philosophical grounding, a medical patient facing death who views the salvageable existence as a personal hell ought to be able to resist medical intervention. This is within the scope of patient autonomy as already accepted in those cases allowing patients to elude the prospective burdens of life as an amputee, or life dependent on a dialysis machine.

Professor Jay Katz, a staunch advocate of informed consent, suggests an interesting limitation on a patient's prerogative to decline life-saving medical treatment. He contends that a competent patient ought to be entitled to reject such treatment even for a "foolish" or "unwise" reason—so long as the patient articulates *some* reason for his decision.[50] If the patient insists on rejecting life-saving treatment "without any explanation," Professor Katz would be inclined to override the patient's determination.

The motivation behind the Katz position is certainly commendable. It is aimed at assuring that the patient's decision is a truly informed one. The physician seeks to know what motivates the patient to make a seemingly unreasoned decision, in order to at least try and confront the patient's objections to treatment.

There can be no quarrel with the effort to engage the patient in careful conversation about his life-rejecting determination. The question is, what follows if the patient persists in his refusal to explain his decision. My own preference would be to respect the patient's choice so long as a conscientious determination can be made—based on the patient's general demeanor and other conversations—that the patient is competent. This would be so even in the rare instance when the patient chooses to cloud his ultimate motivations in silence.

Many physicians cannot brook Professor Katz's basic toleration of the salvageable patient's seemingly "foolish" or "unwise" determination to reject life-preserving treatment. A common strategy in such instances is to make highly strained findings of incompetency in order to justify the medical intervention which the physician strongly favors.[51] That is, the physician will make a determination (based in part on the patient's seemingly aberrational decision to resist treatment) that the patient is incompetent. Life-saving therapy will then be administered. This manipulation of competency is presumably based on well-meaning life-preserving instincts. From a practical point of view, the strategy can succeed so long as a close relative or friend does not take legal steps to protect the patient's choice, and so long as the patient physically cooperates with the administration of treatment. (Of course, some physicians might even be willing to override physical resistance from the patient).

Physicians who thus manipulate findings of incompetency probably feel that they are acting on sound humanitarian grounds, and that the salvageable patient will someday thank them. Sometimes that latter assumption may even be borne out. The story is often told of the burn victim who—severely burned on much of his body and facing excruciating treatment and a prospective existence as a blind and disabled person—sought to reject therapy. Therapy was administered, the patient was saved, and the recovered individual eventually expressed great delight at still being alive.[52]

The manipulation of competency in circumstances of salvageable patients, or even the plain overriding of the salvageable patient's will, is understandable. The impulse to preserve salvageable life is strong. Moreover, the physician does not face a very serious threat of legal liability in such circumstances. Monetary "damages" are nonexistent when a patient has been salvaged to a healthful existence. And it is hard to penalize a medical professional for a good faith effort to preserve human life.

The manipulative practices still constitute a perversion of the principles of autonomy and self-determination which underlie the doctrine of informed consent. The whole basis of this doctrine is to allow individuals to order their own priorities and values and to determine their own medical fates. The prerogative applies even if the patient's judgment is wrong or foolish from an "objective" perspective. The doctrine of informed consent assumes its largest importance when the patient's choice diverges from the physicians' advice. Otherwise, the doctrine diverges from "consent" and merely requires that the patient be "informed" about what the physician has chosen to do. Even the recovered burn victim, happy to be alive, was not convinced that his doctors had acted properly. In 1985, twelve years after his medical ordeal, he commented: "I feel strongly that it is the individual affected, and he alone, that has the right to make such decisions."[53]

Self-Induced Crisis: Prisoners and Handicapped Persons Resisting Nourishment

Efforts have been made to invoke the self-determination prerogative of a terminally ill medical patient in the context of "healthy" persons resisting all nourishment, including medically administered intravenous feeding. This has occurred in two settings. Hunger striking prisoners have sought to resist forced feeding or nourishment ordered by prison authorities. And a physically handicapped individual sought to invoke hospital assistance in the process of starving herself to death. For reasons which will be articulated below, neither of these efforts is congruent with the right of the dying medical patient to refuse life-preserving medical treatment.

Approximately ten courts have faced the issue of the hunger striking prisoner within the last ten years. Only one of them—the Supreme Court of Georgia—upheld the prisoner's effort to resist the administration of nourishment. That case was *Zant v. Prevatte,* decided in 1982.[54] There, the prisoner launched a hunger strike to try and induce his transfer to a prison which he considered to be a safer locale. The Georgia court upheld the prisoner's refusal to allow intrusions on his person, even though such intrusions were calculated to save his life. The court found the prisoner's claim consistent with the right of privacy recognized in cases allowing dying medical patients to refuse life-preserving medical treatment.

Zant stands in lonely isolation. *Von Holden v. Chapman,* a New York case decided in 1982, is representative of the remainder of the courts which have uniformly rejected the claims of hunger-striking prisoners.[55] Mark David Chapman was serving a twenty-year-to-life term for the murder of singer John Lennon. He launched his hunger strike with the expressed intent to starve himself to death in order to draw attention to "the starving children in the world." His fast had lasted twenty-two days when judicial authorization of forced nourishment was sought and granted. The court found the following state interests to prevail over the prisoner's claim: "the obligation of the State to protect the health and welfare of persons in its care and custody, its interest in the preservation of life, and its interest in maintaining rational and orderly procedures in its institutions. . . ."[56] The opinion went on to ridicule the notion that the self-destructive act in issue might be constitutionally protected. The right of a competent patient to refuse life-preserving medical treatment in the face of a "natural degenerative condition" was viewed as dissimilar to the prisoner's asserted right to starve to death.

The remaining courts have sided with the *Chapman* court. It is common in these opinions to note that prisoners possess greatly reduced expectations of privacy compared with the general population. It's also common to rely on an asserted governmental concern with "orderly prison administration."[57] The precise administrative concern is usually not spelled out. Ostensibly, a hunger striking prisoner would present very little burden to a corrections system. He can be relegated to a designated location; periodic observation to ensure humane conditions and to check continued voluntary abstinence doesn't seem like a large drain on the system.

Nonetheless, these cases by and large seem correctly decided. For in most of them the prisoner is using the starvation tactic to try and extort concessions of one form or another from prison administrators. The spectre of the dying supplicant places considerable pressure on the responsible administrator, a form of coercion which shouldn't have to be tolerated. This point is most evident where the prisoner's underlying demand is unlawful, such as a demand for premature release or establishment of segregated facilities. But even if the prisoner's objective is within the discretion of the administrator, the threat to starve to death is an inappropriate form of extortion or coercion within a correctional facility. Of course, not every hunger strike is aimed at extracting some demand. Chapman's fast, for example, was aimed at making a symbolic statement about certain world conditions. Such a case can be resolved along with the case of the handicapped hospital patient, a topic to which I now turn.

Elizabeth Bouvia was a twenty-six-year-old quadriplegic who had suffered from cerebral palsy. She had been left with virtually no motor function in her limbs or skeletal muscles. While she had a life expectancy of fifteen to twenty years, she would always be almost totally dependent on others, a condition which she apparently regarded as "humiliating." In early 1984, she checked into a California hospital with the avowed intention of resisting all nourishment and starving to death. She was mentally competent. Ms. Bouvia apparently felt mired in a severely disabled and personally distasteful existence. While she had previously functioned well despite her handicaps—she had received a college degree and had been married—she had reached a competent determination not to continue living. She sought the hospital's cooperation in providing painkillers and hygienic care to ease the dying process. The hospital objected to Ms. Bouvia's plan and sought judicial guidance. After a protracted hearing, the California court ruled that the hospital need not cooperate with Ms. Bouvia. Nutrition was forcibly administered through a naso-gastric tube until she checked out of the hospital on April 9, 1984.[58]

Ms. Bouvia was seeking to die through starvation not in order to coerce certain conduct from those around her, but simply because she no longer wished to live. Like Mark David Chapman, she lacked an individual's normal resources to accomplish suicide through more mundane channels—she because she was a quadriplegic and he because he was a prisoner. Both also sought to invoke the notion that an adult patient has a right—based either in the Constitution or common law—to resist life-preserving medical treatment. In essence, they argued that the intravenous or other forced administration of nutrition by medical personnel constituted an unwanted form of medical care and bodily invasion which they were entitled to resist.

With all due empathy to Ms. Bouvia's sad plight, I can't conclude that her case is covered by the previously discussed principles governing the handling of dying medical patients. It is true that she is asserting a personal interest in bodily integrity as against government interference. It is also true that her motivation was similar to that of the patients who were previously found entitled to resist life-preserving amputations or dialysis—that is, the avoidance of a prospective existence that is personally intolerable. Nonetheless, the self-induced nature of Ms. Bouvia's "medical" status differentiates her case from the others, at least for constitutional purposes. The constitutionally grounded decisions recognizing patient autonomy and self-determination all involved an independently occurring medical pathology which the patient chose not to resist. The patient and surrounding medical personnel were allowed to "let nature take its course." This traditional deference to informed patient consent does not necessarily carry over to a person who starves himself or herself into a potentially fatal state. In short, this novel form of suicide does not fit comfortably within the bounds of the previously defined privacy interest in rejecting life-preserving medical treatment.

This is not to say that intravenous nourishment is not within the bounds of "medical treatment" which can be resisted by dying medical patients. To the contrary, where artificial nutrition is an adjunct to a general medical effort to thwart a nonpatient-induced pathological condition, it can be regarded as part of a "medical" arsenal. Such nourishment should be deemed withdrawable in circumstances where the full arsenal of medical technology can be withdrawn. This topic will be examined in detail in chapter 2. But where a sound person seeks to induce a terminal condition by starvation, artificial nourishment is no longer part of ancillary medical care arrayed to combat a separate pathological state.

While Ms. Bouvia's case may not fit comfortably within the constitutionally-based framework of a dying medical patient suffering from a natural degenerative condition, this does not mean that as a matter of governmental policy her plea to be allowed to resist nourishment ought to be spurned. So long as her starvation is not extortionate in form (as in the prisoner cases) my inclination would be to respect her self-determination even in this unusual format. The resort to her technique will almost surely be an extraordinarily rare event. Most people who seriously desire self-destruction have a variety of devices—pills and poisons—available. She, as a quadriplegic, lacked this normal access to self-destructive tools and was reduced to this excruciatingly inefficient technique. Her isolated effort to resist nourishment poses no significant threat to material governmental interests.

Of course, Ms. Bouvia was seeking to enlist medical assistance in her self-destructive act. That fact has some implications. Patients have no right to impose on physicians' scruples in dictating the course of medical handling. Many physicians may have principled objections to participating in what they perceive of as an unnatural self-destructive act by a salvageable individual. They can't be forced to cooperate. Their proper course is to withdraw from the case and allow the patient to seek medical personnel who can, in good conscience, follow the patient's bidding. In point of fact, testimony in the *Bouvia* proceeding indicated that some medical personnel could, consistent with their consciences, cooperate in her effort to resist nutrition.

The better course then, even if not constitutionally mandated, is not to impose the physician's will on the competent patient resisting nutrition, at least not outside of the prison setting. Within the prison setting, prisoners should not be able to extort demands through starvation. However, in the rare case (like Chapman's) where the prisoner seeks no return from administrative personnel, other than to be allowed to resist nourishment, I would allow a competent prisoner to reject such nourishment.

Obviously, my position on starvation cases runs counter to traditional notions regarding suicide and suicide prevention. I will explain how I resolve these tensions in Chapter 2.

II

DISPELLING THE MYTHS

The volitional taking of human life normally implicates the law of homicide. As a consequence, concerns about criminal liability surfaced early on in discussions about terminating or withholding medical treatment from dying patients. At first blush, these concerns seemed warranted. Intentional conduct which appreciably shortens another person's life generally constitutes homicide, an unlawful killing. Safeguarding of human life has traditionally been deemed a preeminent value, and equality of life has been regarded as a cornerstone of the administration of law. A gravely ill person would therefore be protected just as a healthy and vigorous one.

Altruistic motive—a desire to relieve another person's suffering—would not constitute a defense for an intentional killing. Mercy killing is regarded as homicide, even though juries frequently sympathize with the killer and either acquit outright or convict of offenses which will entail light punishment.

Nor would specific intent to cause death be a necessary element in a homicide prosecution. Normally it is enough that the actor knows that death will ensue from his or her action; the actor is presumed to intend the natural consequences of the act. A physician who removes a respirator or an I.V. knows that the moment of death will be accelerated by his or her action.

Consent of the patient would not necessarily matter. A person cannot lawfully consent to homicide. And even passive handling of a dying patient at the request of the patient risks a finding of aiding and abetting suicide, or so it would seem.

Commentators struggle to find bases on which to differentiate humane termination of medical care from unlawful killing. Discussion has focussed on possible distinctions between "commission" and "omission," or between "extraordinary" and "ordinary" forms of medical treatment. The cases mentioned in chapter 1 have shown that common sense and flexibility in the judicial evolution of legal doctrine are better guides than the fine technical distinctions suggested by commentators. Judges have been able to endorse humane medical practices, especially those respecting decisions of competent patients, without reliance on the arcane lines originally suggested.

The Omission-Commission Dichotomy

Law has traditionally refrained from imposing either criminal or civil liability on a person for failure to save or rescue a dying individual—as opposed to affirmatively acting to terminate another's existence, which is homicide. The approach was not formulated with the handling of medical patients in mind, but reflected general reluctance to impose an affirmative obligation on one citizen toward another, as well as difficulty in determining what quantity of affirmative effort might reasonably be demanded from people.

Since withholding of life-preserving medical care was clearly passive behavior, an omission, it was initially thought that law might latch onto this factor to approve humane decisions to allow terminally ill patients to expire without unwanted or excessive medical intervention. A common approach was to refer to medical omission as "letting nature take its course"—with the implication that any ensuing death would be attributable to natural causes rather than physician conduct, thus absolving the physician from responsibility. A physician who fails to place an expiring patient on a respirator could be viewed as behaving passively—omitting life-sustaining machinery—even though the material consequence might be the death of the patient earlier than would otherwise be the case.

The omission-commission dichotomy has a long history in moral philosophy. And it has a venerable place in portions of both criminal and tort law. But this active/passive distinction was, from the start, too simplistic to shape legal liability in the context of dying medical patients. Disconnecting a respirator clearly entailed affirmative conduct. Yet, from the perspective of morals and common sense, withdrawal of a respirator could not be distinguished from failing to start the machinery, or from allowing an oxygen supply to run out without replacement, both being passive omissions.

The courts have been flexible enough to recognize the absence of a critical distinction between withholding medical procedures from terminally ill patients and terminating such procedures once instituted. In *Barber v. Superior Court,*[1] a California court recently acknowledged that withdrawal of an intravenous tube should be regarded as equivalent to withholding the procedure for purposes of assessing physicians' liability. The New Jersey Supreme Court, in January 1985, adopted an identical position toward removal of a naso-gastric tube from a moribund patient.[2] Similarly, the Florida court in *Satz v. Perlmutter*,[3] refused to draw a determinative distinction between disconnection of a respirator and failure to institute the procedure at all. If withholding of the medical procedure could legally be justified, so could termination of the procedure.

In both withholding and terminating medical care from a moribund patient, the determinative legal factor is not passive "omission," but rather the bounds of the service obligation flowing from doctor to patient. That is, a doctor who omits life-preserving measures in a situation where such measures are demanded by professional norms risks civil and criminal liability despite the passive nature of his conduct. By contrast, the physician who actively "pulls the plug" and precipitates death is free from liability so long as he is following professional norms which are also acceptable to the general society (as reflected by legislatures and courts).

The doctor/patient relationship is understood to be a fiduciary relationship whose terms are largely implied by law. The bounds of the physician's obligations are seldom bargained out in explicit terms. The implied terms or bounds are largely shaped by evolving norms of the medical profession itself, so long as those norms are sufficiently humane and sensitive to avoid societal censure via legislatures or courts. (The courts do not *have* to acquiesce in medical practices surrounding the delicate matter of preservation of life. At any point that medical practices are deemed to violate reasonable fiduciary limits—normally meaning that a physician's conduct must be consistent with the best interests of the patient—there is a possibility of judicial intervention.)

With regard to medical practices involving active termination of previously instituted treatment measures, there has thus far been no clash between medical norms and judicial sources asked to validate such norms. Medical practice in the case of competent, terminally ill patients[4] has evolved toward concern for the dying patient's self-defined suffering, and easing of the patient's dying process. This has come to mean adherence to a competent, terminally ill patient's requests regarding the nature of treatment to be administered. This approach has been increasingly applied whether the decision involves detachment of medical equipment or nonattachment of such equipment. These medical trends have effectively gained endorsement from the judiciary. The judicial decisions described in chapter 1 acknowledge that emerging medical practices of shaping care in accordance with a dying patient's wishes are consistent with societal respect for individual autonomy in shaping the dying process. Cases like *Barber* and *Conroy* recognize that active termination of treatment can be viewed from a legal perspective in the same fashion as the withholding of treatment.

All this does not mean that the omission-commission dichotomy has no relevance to the context of the dying medical patient. Active euthanasia—in the form, say, of lethal injections—has never been endorsed in the United States. Active intervention through external agents, such as poisons, can be differentiated, for legal purposes, from "active" termination of previously started medical procedures. Nor does the endorsement of medical withdrawal of life-preserving care on the ground of a patient's desire to avoid excessive suffering mean that active euthanasia on the same ground must eventually be endorsed.

The impetus for affirmative acts of voluntary euthanasia stems largely from the same concerns underlying respect for a patient's refusal of life-preserving treatment—that is, providing relief for a patient suffering the indignities of a terminal illness, and respect for patient self-determination. Nonetheless, there are distinctions. Most people feel an instinctive aversion to allowing administration of lethal agents, while removal of medical equipment does not evoke the same negative response. Furthermore, withholding of further medical care results, in some instances, in the moribund patient remaining alive for some period, with a resulting opportunity to change one's mind and request continued medical intervention. During that same period, there may also be a continuing possibility of remission. Administration of a lethal agent, by contrast, leaves no such possibilities.

More importantly, it is not clear whether with emerging acceptance of a patient's right to decline treatment, there would be a strong utility to active euthanasia. By declining life-preserving care, the patient can precipitate death. In the vast majority of cases, analgesics and sedatives will mitigate the suffering which would accompany any protracted terminal stages. Where pain or other suffering is unmitigated, a possibility exists of resisting nutrition as part of the rejection of life-preserving medical intervention—a topic which will be discussed below. In short, active euthanasia is not necessarily a logical or necessary sequel to recognition of a patient's prerogative to resist life-preserving medical treatment.

The line between active euthanasia and "allowing the patient to die" is not always self-evident. I've cited as one example the removal of medical equipment previously instituted. The line between manipulation of medical equipment and active administration of death is even more blurred with respect to the occasional medical practice of administering pain-killing narcotics which also accelerate the death of the terminally ill recipient. This is commonly regarded as legally unassailable even though it constitutes a willful intervention done with knowledge of the inevitable fatal consequence. The "moral" explanation is that there is a "double effect" from the physician's act, with pain relief being the primary, intended consequence and accelerated death a secondary consequence.

This "double effect" rationale has been sufficient to satisfy religious and moral philosophers. But that rationale does not satisfactorily account for the law's acquiescence in the practice. From a legal perspective, the narcotic administration might technically be regarded as homicide, at least if life is appreciably shortened. Neither the fact that the actor's (doctor's) motive is commendable (relief of pain) nor that the recipient of the injection consents would normally relieve the actor of legal responsibility for the life-shortening deed. To offer an analogy, a defendant who bodily whipped another person would not legally be absolved of the crime of "maiming" or "infliction of bodily injury" on the basis that the "victim" was a person who both consented to the whipping and derived great masochistic pleasure from the event.

The act of narcotic administration goes unchallenged in legal fora simply because of universal moral acceptance of its propriety, if not necessity. There is a tacit understanding that prosecution would never be undertaken, even if the causal connection between the analgesic and death could be established. In this matter, as in the case of actively "pulling a plug" or otherwise removing a respirator, medical practice has won de facto legal acceptance because of widespread acknowledgement of its humane grounding.

Extraordinary versus Ordinary Procedures

In the fifties and sixties, the notion that life-preserving medical procedures could legally be withheld or withdrawn from a terminally ill patient was novel and startling. Perhaps as a means of cushioning the shock effect from that notion, early proponents frequently adopted a limitation first expressed in Catholic moral theology—that only "extraordinary" means of care could be foregone. Many of the judicial opinions on the subject of death and dying, including most of the cases discussed in chapter 1, continue to mouth this formula while neither analyzing its meaning nor applying its limitation. The formula itself is confusing and unhelpful and ought to be discarded entirely. In the context of competent patients, a terminally ill person is entitled to determine which medical interventions will be undertaken during his dying process—whether "extraordinary" in some sense or not. And even in the context of an incompetent patient, the extraordinary-ordinary dichotomy yields more heat than light.

The term "extraordinary" medical treatment potentially includes a wide range of factors. The term instinctively evokes notions of novelty and complexity—an artificial heart or heart transplant, to cite extreme examples. Expense might also be part of extraordinariness. In fact, the Catholic concept does include cost of treatment as a relevant factor. Burdensomeness to the patient—in terms of pain or intrusiveness of the procedure—might also be relevant. Usefulness to the patient—in terms of the duration and quality of the existence to be salvaged by the procedure—might be relevant, depending on who is defining "extraordinary." Thus, the term "extraordinary," by itself, does little to pinpoint the variables, let alone explain the relationship among them.

Many writers have recognized that the appropriateness of a particular medical intervention must be fixed in accord with the patient's condition and prognosis. The "quality" of remaining existence—in terms of benefits and burdens to the patient—rather than complexity or novelty of proposed treatment becomes the principal determinant of what is appropriate or "extraordinary" (to the extent that this latter term is retained at all). Of course, as to the competent patient, that patient's own assessment of his status and prospects are largely determinative of what is "extraordinary." The recent President's Commission for the study of ethical problems in medicine confirmed this approach. In that group's view, "extraordinary treatment is that which, in the patient's view, entails significantly greater burdens than benefits and is therefore undesirable. . . ."[5] (That group also stressed the lack of utility of the term "extraordinary" and suggested abandoning it). Similarly, the blood transfusion, amputation, and dialysis cases discussed in chapter 1 point toward the conclusion that patient assessment of the quality of remaining existence is much more important than the complexity, novelty or expense of life-preserving care whose maintenance is being resisted by the patient.

The New Jersey Supreme Court's 1985 decision in the *Conroy* case represents a major advance in disposing of the "extraordinary-ordinary" dichotomy. As noted, that decision addressed removal of a naso-gastric feeding tube from a semi-comatose, dying patient. In response to the claim that only "extraordinary" means could be omitted from treatment of a dying individual, the court observed that the term extraordinary "has too many conflicting meanings to remain useful."[6] This conclusion flowed from awareness that extraordinariness can be variously predicated on novelty, complexity, expense, invasiveness, painfulness, or utility to the patient. The *Conroy* opinion therefore branded the extraordinary-ordinary distinction "unpersuasive," and added: "To draw a line on this basis for determining whether treatment should be given leads to a semantical milieu that does not advance the analysis."[7] Hopefully, this forceful judicial expression by a respected state supreme court will help give the extraordinariness doctrine the burial it deserves.

For those jurisdictions which don't abandon the extraordinary-ordinary dichotomy, they will at least have to acknowledge the relation between condition of the patient and "extraordinariness" of care. The main consequence of recognizing this relation is to accept that rather routine medical procedures can sometimes be withdrawn. At the very least, these include such simple measures as blood transfusions, basic chemotherapy such as antibiotics, and chest massage or artificial respiration (as part of cardiopulmonary resuscitation). In practice, it is common for physicians to withhold antibiotics from patients in advanced stages of terminal illness in order to permit pneumonia, "the old man's friend," to end the dying process. A 1979 report in the New England Journal of Medicine describes, for example, how antibiotic therapy was omitted in numerous cases of terminal cancer patients suffering during a protracted demise in an extended care facility.[8]

Medical commentary has also acknowledged the practice of issuing "no-code" or "do not resuscitate" (DNR) orders on some hospitalized patients' charts—instructions that in the event of heart stoppage, cardiovascular resuscitation is not to be undertaken. The primary issue regarding DNR orders is not whether a particular resuscitory technique is extraordinary or ordinary in nature, but whether any effort to revive the expiring patient is called for. Indeed, the biggest question regarding DNR is over the process to be followed in issuing such orders, and over adherence to the patient's prerogatives. Traditional notions of informed consent dictate that a competent patient must authorize any such order. But medical personnel, not surprisingly, are reluctant to raise an issue about a prospective traumatic event that isn't immediately pressing and indeed may never occur. There are indications that doctors sometimes rely on "tacit understandings" with patients in situations where no pointed discussions have been held and where the patient's actual position differs from the doctor's assumption about the patient's preferences.[9]

There is every reason to think that courts will continue to acquiesce to the notion that even simplistic medical procedures may be foregone where the patient's condition, prognosis and wishes so warrant. As noted, numerous decisions have upheld refusals of life-preserving blood transfusions. One Massachusetts decision has endorsed entry of a no resuscitation order for a highly debilitated, terminally ill patient.[10] A particularly insightful California judge recently noted that the ordinary-extraordinary dichotomy "begs the question." He went on to note that the critical issue in withdrawal of medical care from the critically ill (incompetent patient) should be "whether the proposed treatment is proportionate or disproportionate in terms of the benefits to be gained versus the burdens caused."[11] This effectively meant that simplistic procedures could be withdrawn, even from an incompetent patient, if the patient's prognosis was sufficiently dismal. (In that particular case, to be discussed below, an intravenous feeding tube was removed from a comatose patient.)

Non-Feeding as Withdrawal of Medical Therapy

Both medical practice and judicial response indicate that a wide range of medical procedures can be withdrawn in order to ease the dying process for a terminally ill individual. The reported cases have most commonly dealt with measures that are indisputably "medical" in nature—such as blood transfusions, respirators, chemotherapy, or dialysis. An emerging issue is whether nutrition—through intravenous tubes (I.V.), naso-gastric tubes, or even basic oral administration—can sometimes be withdrawn from the terminally ill.

A common instinctive reaction to the issue is to regard nutrition as natural "sustenance" rather than medical treatment. Many religious commentators, whether of Catholic or orthodox Jewish persuasion, adopt this approach. The implication is that nutrition is outside the area of "medical" procedures which might conceivably be withheld from a terminally ill patient. An alternative view—one that I'm inclined to endorse—regards nutrition as a medical procedure where it is part of a program sustaining the existence of a patient threatened by pathology. A third view is that "artificial nutrition"—nourishment administered by medical personnel through injections or implantation of tubes as opposed to oral ingestion of food—can be regarded as a medical procedure.

Normally, feeding is considered part of the palliative care administered by hospital staff to a dying patient in order to promote that patient's comfort. This category of care would include, besides feeding—administration of analgesics and/or sedation, easing of body position, and provision of a clean and warm environment. But at least where associated with underlying pathology which irrevocably fixes the demise of the patient, nutrition might arguably be classified as part of the medical framework potentially removable according to customary criteria—adherence to the patient's desires or to the humane easing of the dying process. This classification is most natural in reference to nutritive processes which are obviously medical in nature—for example, surgical removal of blockages to food passages or surgical implantation of nutrition tubes where natural alimentation processes aren't functioning. Yet even routinely inserted naso-gastric tubes, or intravenous lines, or even hand-feeding might be deemed terminable in order to ease the dying process for a patient who is afflicted with a terminal illness and has made a determination that the potential suffering from further treatment and/or associated effects of the dying process are so distasteful that he or she prefers to expire without further medical intervention. Palliative care of the dying patient, including nutrition, bathing, etc., should be handled according to the competent patient's preferences, just as more complex medical procedures such as chemotherapy or a respirator would be handled.

The arguments against treating nutrition and hydration as part of the medical framework surrounding patients are generally unpersuasive. One claim is that withdrawal of nutrition hastens death, and thus is incompatible with the physician's customary role of striving to preserve life. But the tension between withdrawal of nutrition and the medical role would appear to be little different from the similar tension when machinery is stopped, chemotherapy is foregone, or resuscitation procedures are omitted—all with the object of easing the dying process or adhering to the patient's instructions.

A second claim is that feeding has a special symbolic significance which differentiates it from other aspects of handling dying patients. Feeding a helpless individual normally connotes sharing and compassion. According to Daniel Callahan, it is "the perfect symbol of the fact that human life is inescapably social and communal."[12]

The altruism embodied in feeding seems little different from the altruism normally involved in furnishing antibiotics, blood transfusions, medicines, or chest massage—all of them simplistic, relatively non-intrusive procedures which may be foregone pursuant to the instructions of a terminally ill patient. On occasion, feeding or nutrition may carry with it no benefit to the patient, or may even prolong a torturous dying process, and thus lose its usual symbolic cast. The question becomes not whether nutrition can ever be omitted, but under what circumstances such omissions are ethically and legally permissible.

A third objection to viewing the withholding of nutrition as equivalent to the withholding of other medical treatment is that the cause of death becomes starvation (or dehydration) rather than simply allowing a fatal disease process to run its course. The charge is that a patient is "dehydrated" to death, rather than death occurring from natural causes.[13] This charge has no force where the nutrition withheld is "artificial nutrition" (I.V., naso-gastric tube, etc.) necessitated by pathology (such as a blockage in the esophagus or intestines). In those instances, if artificial nutrition is withdrawn or withheld pathological conditions will simply be allowed to run their natural course. Similarly, for the terminally ill patient who is so deteriorated that the swallowing reflex has been lost, as for the patient whose medical pathology prevents oral taking of nourishment, artificial nutrition represents interference with a "natural" decline—just as a respirator does for a patient who can no longer breathe independently. Yet no one argues that a patient is improperly being "choked" to death if a respirator is removed pursuant to a terminal patient's request to be allowed to die. The question in each case is the scope of a patient's prerogative to determine the course of the dying process, and the corresponding obligations of medical personnel.

The independent causation argument (death is caused by dehydration rather than disease) has more force where oral feeding is physically possible. Even there, nutrition might be viewed as simply part of the palliative care being administered to a patient otherwise being treated during a fatal disease process. If the patient is entitled to reject a variety of purely medical treatments and thus provoke death, it may well be humane and sound to permit rejection of nutrition. A terminally ill patient's refusal to eat would not seem very different from a terminally ill patient rejecting antibiotics with the knowledge that an infection will soon set in and the patient will die from the infection. Permitting death by starvation or dehydration may well be humane in the sense that any associated discomfort may well be less than the pain accompanying the dying process if that process is allowed to run its course.[14] Moreover, forced feeding of a dying patient who chooses to resist nutrition might well be viewed as a disturbing affront to that patient's dignity. Legal permissibility of withholding nutrition should hinge not on the precise cause of death on the medical certificate (whether dehydration or cancer), but on the scope of the affirmative obligations owed to a dying patient by surrounding medical personnel.

The question remains how much support the view of feeding as medical therapy can garner in the legal arena. The cases described in chapter 1 demonstrate widespread and growing medical and judicial recognition that individual autonomy and self-determination entitle a competent patient to shape the dying process, even if that means rejection of procedures which could forestall death. This principle, which allows the patient to determine when the burdens of the dying process outweigh the benefits of life-preserving measures, seems fully applicable to the matter of nutrition and hydration. A recent Presidential Commission report, in accepting this principle, specifically noted its applicability to such simplistic procedures as blood transfusions, administration of antibiotics, and "parenteral nutrition and hydration."[15] A 1984 article by medical figures from several eminent teaching centers also acknowledged that hydration and nutrition may be withheld from patients in the terminal phase of an irreversible illness, at least where consistent with a patient's comfort and wishes.[16]

Judicial authority is likely to accept and endorse this medical recognition of a terminally ill patient's prerogative to resist nutrition. For the courts will be guided in this area, in the absence of legislative direction,[17] by sensitive and humane medical practices. That is, if medical authorities widely adopt the view that nutrition is part of the array of medical interventions surrounding terminal care, the chances of judicial acceptance of the position will be enhanced.

To date, though, there has been very little judicial treatment of the precise issue. As noted in chapter 1, a lower court in New York refused to intervene when an eighty-five-year-old former college president, suffering from the effects of a disabling stroke, resisted nutrition and starved himself to death.[18] And one court has even allowed hunger-striking prisoners to resist feeding—an extension of self-determination well beyond the context of the terminally ill medical patient.[19] Such a court would presumably endorse patients' resistance to nutrition in the context of a patient's shaping of an inexorable dying process.

The bulk of the judicial discussion of nutrition as part of medical therapy has come in the context of several cases involving incompetent patients. One clear expression of judicial willingness to regard nutrition as part of the medical framework surrounding the dying patient came in a 1983 California case, *Barber v. Superior Court.*[20] In *Barber,* an intermediate appellate court rejected efforts to prosecute physicians who, pursuant to a family's request, had removed intravenous tubes providing nutrition and hydration to a permanently comatose patient. The patient had previously lapsed into "an indefinite vegetative existence" without any higher cognitive brain function. At first, the family requested removal of all machines sustaining life, including a respirator. When the patient continued to breathe, the family asked that he not be disturbed at all. After two days of deliberation, the responsible physicians complied and ordered removal of the tubes providing hydration and nourishment, thus precipitating death. When local authorities initiated criminal prosecution, the physicians sought a judicial declaration that their conduct had been lawful. A lower court initially ruled that their conduct did ostensibly involve homicide, but an appellate court reversed the decision.

The appellate court ruled that despite "the emotional symbolism" of feeding, artificial nutrition could, in the context of a permanently co-matose patient, be addressed like other medically administered life support procedures. That is, the benefits and burdens of each procedure could be assessed, and any process could be withdrawn where it was of no net benefit to the patient. The court observed:

> Medical procedures to provide nutrition and hydration are more similar to other medical procedures than to typical human ways of providing nutrition and hydration. Their benefits and burdens ought to be evaluated in the same manner as any other medical procedure.[21]

The basis for this conclusion—that nutrition could legitimately be withdrawn from a permanently comatose patient—was laid in the classic *Quinlan* case. There, the New Jersey Supreme Court authorized removal of a respirator from a twenty-two-year-old in a "persistent vegetative state," with the expectation that the comatose woman would soon die. In *Quinlan*, removal of the naso-gastric feeding tube and of antibiotic administration were not specifically addressed; the patient's guardian was guided by a religious precept that such simple measures were "ordinary" and therefore not expendable under any circumstances. But the guiding principles set down by the court with respect to the respirator would seem to permit withdrawal of such measures as antibiotic and nutrition administration. As to both a respirator and a naso-gastric tube, the permanently comatose patient would not be deemed to benefit from continuation of the procedures and, the patient being insensate, could not suffer from their removal. Humane medical practice—a consideration valued by the court—would then permit removal of all artificial interventions sustaining such a marginal and dismal existence.

In January 1985, in the *Conroy* case,[22] the New Jersey Supreme Court followed up on the groundwork laid in *Quinlan*. That court ruled that "artificial feedings" such as naso-gastric tubes, gastrostomies, and intravenous infusions are "medical procedures" potentially withdrawable from a dying patient according to standards applied to other forms of medical treatment. That ruling came in the context of an effort to remove a naso-gastric tube sustaining an eighty-four-year-old woman, bedridden, virtually insensate, and afflicted with a variety of fatal conditions including heart disease and diabetes. Her nephew, as guardian, sought judicial authorization to have the naso-gastric tube removed so that Ms. Conroy could be allowed to die from starvation within a few days. Otherwise, the projection was that she could languish for months or even a year. In response to the hospital's contention that provision of basic nutrition is categorically different from medical treatment such as a respirator, the court commented:

> Analytically, artificial feeding by means of a nasogastric tube or intra-
> venous infusion can be seen as equivalent to artificial breathing by means
> of a respirator. Both prolong life through mechanical means when the
> body is no longer able to perform a vital bodily function on its own.[23]

Justice Schreiber's opinion added: "A competent patient has the right to decline any medical treatment, including artificial feeding, and should retain that right when and if he becomes incompetent."[24]

While I would go further and include manual feeding as a procedure potentially withholdable at the patient's request (even though the patient is still physically capable of normal ingestion and digestion), the *Conroy* opinion is a major step forward. Presumably, it will greatly influence subsequent judicial decisions as did the *Quinlan* case before it. *Conroy,* an expression by New Jersey's highest state court, reinforces the conclusion previously reached by intermediate appellate courts in California and Massachusetts,[25] that artificial feeding can be regarded as part of the medical procedures potentially terminable in the context of a dying patient.

Conroy also raises, in stark terms, the difficult issue of how to handle incompetent patients in chronic, degenerative states who are not facing immediately life-threatening conditions. (The patient there was pro-jected to live for as long as a year if nutrition were maintained.) The question is not just nourishment. Nonresuscitation orders will inevitably be an issue, and continuation of antibiotics and other measures to fore-stall life-threatening conditions must be addressed. These questions are part of the larger problem of how to handle the incompetent, terminally ill patient. I'll address that whole matter, including who can make deci-sions and according to what criteria, in chapters 3 and 4. My point here is simply that—at the very least where the moribund patient is competent to make his or her own decisions surrounding the dying process— artificial nutrition can be regarded as part of the general range of medical decisions and handled according to the same criteria as other medical interventions (as to which patient autonomy plays a predomi-nant role).

Death sometimes comes to a geriatric patient after a slow and gentle decline, ending with a few hours of terminal bronchopneumonia with the patient in coma. But in other instances, the dying process can be extremely distressful. This may be so for end stage renal disease, respira-tory failure, or cancer, as examples. The end may come hard for a chronic emphysema sufferer, unable to speak because of a tracheotomy and tortured by breathing difficulty or paroxysms of cough. For these latter classes of patient, the prospect of rejecting further nutrition (as well as other life-preserving measures) would seem to offer welcome relief.

Up to this point, discussion has focussed on nutrition as a form of medical intervention during the last stages of a terminal illness. The naso-gastric tube or intravenous line, it is suggested, is then just part of the variety of medical paraphenalia potentially removable from the patient. For some patients suffering from chronic degenerative diseases, such as Alzheimer's disease, death may come after a torturous process of deterioration, loss of faculties, and agonizing suffering. I respectfully suggest that for these chronic disease sufferers, as well, nutrition can be regarded as an essentially medical process terminable at the request of the competent patient. That is, even before a terminal stage at which death is imminent, the patient facing a torturous and inexorable decline ought to be able to repudiate nutrition just as he or she might repudiate further chemotherapy or a respirator. In short, imminence of death should not be a prerequisite to a terminally ill patient's prerogative to reject nutrition any more than it would be a precondition to the rejection of more complex therapy. This is consistent with the position adopted in chapter 1 that the autonomy accorded a dying medical patient includes the prerogative to decide when the projected existence is so dismal that further intervention may be rejected.

The reported cases in which patients were in effect allowed to acceler- ate a nonimminent death usually entailed rejection of physically invasive procedures—amputations, or dialysis treatments. But I submit that less invasive procedures—such as blood transfusions, or cardiopulmonary resuscitation, or antibiotics—can also be foregone by the dying patient. As to nutrition, if the patient can find medical personnel who, in good conscience, will cooperate with the patient's decision to forego feeding even though death is not yet imminent, that rejection too should be permissible. Thus, as noted, the evolving attitudes of physicians will play a large role in shaping ultimate judicial approaches.

As mentioned above, I would go even further than the *Conroy* case and support rejection of manual feeding (not just artificial nutrition) by a competent medical patient. That is, even when the terminally ill patient's physical condition doesn't necessitate artifical nourishment and the pa- tient has been receiving oral feeding, the patient should have the pre- rogative to reject all nutrition including oral feeding—at least where the patient's condition is such that a request to forego further medical treatment would be honored.[26]

A poignant example of the kind of case in which a competent, chron- ically ill person should be permitted to resist nutrition arose in 1984 in New York.[27] The individual in question was a fifty-four-year-old woman who, until a tragic fall in 1982, had been a vigorous and active person. She was the devoted mother of five children, three of them married, a fourth in college, and the fifth a fifteen-year-old living at home. The tragic fall in 1982 fractured vertebrae and left the woman a total quadriplegic. She was unable to move her hands, feet, arms, or legs. She was incontinent, and unable to breathe on her own. A mechanical ventilator pumped air into her lungs via an opening made in the trachea.

The woman petitioned a court for a declaratory judgment that, in the event she were again hospitalized (as was frequently the case), she could take only such nourishment as she wished, and that palliative care (pain killers or sedatives) would be administered pursuant to her request. In effect, she wanted confirmation that she would be permitted to starve to death. (For reasons not made clear in the court's opinion, the petitioner was not asking that the ventilator be withdrawn, though she had resisted it in the past.)

The New York court ducked the basic question regarding feeding. The decision was that the legal controversy was not yet ripe for judicial intervention because the woman was not yet hospitalized. But the judge hinted that the woman's petition would be granted, and her self-determination honored, if a controversy arose after she was hospitalized.

This anonymous woman's situation illustrates why I would classify feeding as a medical procedure—potentially withdrawable at the instigation of a patient—where nutrition is part of an overall medical program sustaining the life of a patient whose life is threatened by independent pathology. Otherwise, a patient may be needlessly condemned to linger in a protracted, distasteful dying process. The other solution—active euthanasia—carries disadvantages (previously detailed) which don't exist in the case of resistance to nutrition.

Of course, a patient's decision to forego a simplistic medical intervention which would significantly prolong his existence—whether a blood transfusion or a naso-gastric feeding tube—brings into play two more myths. The first is that rejection of life-preserving medical treatment constitutes suicide, so that cooperating medical personnel might be implicated in aiding or abetting suicide. The second is that quality of life considerations can and ought to be foreclosed from the medical setting. These notions will be addressed now in turn.

Suicide and Refusals of Treatment

Because the rejection of life-preserving medical treatment entails a form of self-destruction—a voluntary step undertaken with knowledge that death will result—it evokes the spectre of suicide. Suicide, in turn, has traditionally been anathema in Judaeo-Christian culture, prompting both popular condemnation and legal intervention. In the religious sphere, the revulsion toward suicide is grounded primarily on the Sixth Commandment and the belief that only a divinity can control the withdrawal of life. Beyond the religious realm, the English common law attached both criminal and civil penalties to suicide or attempted suicide. Suicide was viewed as an offense against nature, violating instincts of self-preservation, as well as an offense against God, society, and the king. Western culture commonly deems self-destruction to be contrary to man's natural inclinations, a deprivation to society of a person's productive capacity, an evil example to others, and even a rude expression of contempt for society. To the extent that a particular instance of self-destruction may reflect a judgment that "life is not worth living," there is concern that the act may undermine customary reverence for the value of human life.

American law has generally ceased to criminalize suicide or attempted suicide, recognizing that deterrence and punishment are not meaningful concepts in this context. But a variety of common legal provisions still reflect continued societal concern over the phenomenon of suicide. Prohibitions widely exist against "aiding and abetting" suicide, persons are often hospitalized for psychiatric scrutiny after a suicide attempt, and bystanders are authorized to use force necessary to thwart a person about to commit suicide.

Some commentators have argued that refusal of life-preserving medical treatment is tantamount to suicide. It is important, then, to reconcile judicial acquiescence in refusal of treatment with traditional efforts of the legal system to prevent suicide.

At a technical level, there are bases to distinguish refusal of life-preserving medical treatment from "suicide" as defined by law. Suicide commonly means a self-destructive course of conduct calculated to cause the actor's demise. Traditionally, two elements have been included in the legal definition—a self-initiated action, and a specific intention to bring about death.

Courts sympathetic with a patient's prerogative to refuse life-preserving medical treatment have been prone to find both elements lacking in a dying patient's rejection of treatment. Thus, in *Satz v. Perlmutter*,[28] in endorsing a terminally ill patient's request for withdrawal of a respirator, the court pointed out both that the patient had a "basic wish to live" and that ensuing death would be the product of natural afflictions rather than a self-induced agent. Both traditional elements of suicide—self-initiated action and specific intent—were found lacking. The court thereby summarily dismissed any contention that termination of the life-preserving machinery at the patient's request would implicate medical practitioners in a suicide. Other courts have used similar rationales to avoid confronting the common societal aversion to suicide.

These technical differentiations between suicide and the refusal of treatment are only partially convincing. To be sure, specific intent to die is an integral element in the definition of suicide. And mere knowledge that death will ensue from the person's course of conduct is not enough to form specific intent to die. The law has never wished to label as a suicide the person who jumps in front of a car to save another, or who undertakes a heroic, but mortally dangerous military mission. Thus, the courts are correct in asserting that "suicide" requires a finding of specific intent to die. But the specific intent of a terminally ill patient rejecting life-preserving treatment is not always so easy to label.

If the patient is motivated by religious tenets in rejecting treatment—such as the Jehovah's Witness refusing a blood transfusion—then it is usually easy to conclude that there is no specific intent to die. That patient typically has no wish to die, hopes and expects a healing to take place, and is merely adhering to a religious injunction in rejecting the particular treatment at hand. Similarly, the patient who finds a particular medical procedure distasteful—such as an amputation—may have a specific intention to continue living despite the repudiation of one form of therapy.

The specific intent of a terminally ill patient seeking to avoid a prolonged and agonizing dying process is more elusive to define. Though the patient may not wish to die, if the main object is relief from suffering and that object can be attained only by death, then the rejection of further treatment in order to accelerate death is close to the specific intent of any suicide who finds existence painful or meaningless.

The action-inaction dichotomy in this context is also only partially convincing. Certainly, suicide is typically accomplished by affirmative acts such as swallowing poison, shooting oneself, or slitting one's wrists. Refusal of life-preserving treatment qualifies as passive behavior. Nonetheless, it's plausible that the person who refuses to move from the path of an avalanche, or who refuses to swim when tossed into deep water, is committing suicide. The hunger striker who rejects nutrition with the intention of becoming a martyr or making a political statement has many of the attributes of a suicide. Thus, the passive nature of the medical patient's conduct is not a fully satisfying explanation for the reluctance to classify his or her behavior as suicide.

The reality is that over the past twenty years both popular and judicial perceptions have simply come to regard the terminally ill patient's decision regarding how to direct medical intervention in order to shape the dying process as a decision reserved to the patient, and a decision to be deemed outside the realm of suicide. Relief from medical intervention in the face of an inexorable dying process has been accepted as a legitimate form of self-determination. There has been, as described in chapter 1, a confluence in this area of two threads relating to individual autonomy. The first was the traditional notion that a medical patient controls the course of therapy—the doctrine of informed consent that is at the heart of the doctor-patient relationship. The second notion, which emerged with the realization that modern medical technology could preserve patients long beyond the point at which in previous eras they would have died, holds that at least where a patient faces an inexorable death (i.e., is irreversibly terminally ill) there is a patient prerogative to determine how and if to resist the onslaught.

The popular acceptance of these principles has been reflected in several ways. The clearest manifestation was the emergence of a "right to die" or "death with dignity" movement. A further expression was the adoption in numerous state legislatures of so-called living will statutes. Many of these measures explicitly provide that death ensuing from the patient's rejection of life-preserving treatment (pursuant to such statutes) is not to be deemed "suicide." In ecclesiastical circles, a 1980 Vatican statement has explicitly recognized that resistance to "burdensome" medical technology is "not the equivalent of suicide," but rather "an acceptance of the human condition. . . ."[29] In medical circles, focus on the prerogatives of the terminally ill began with extensive literature on how to handle terminally ill patients in the early 1960's and has continued to the present in discussions of hospital ethics committees and the like. It has been clear in all these discussions that physicians did not necessarily equate patient rejection of life-preserving treatment with suicide.

The courts have generally adopted this popular view that a dying patient's resistance to life-preserving treatment constitutes a legitimate form of self-determination taking it outside the realm of suicide. This judicial recognition of patient autonomy is sometimes grounded on a constitutional "privacy right" of the patient, sometimes on a common law right to bodily integrity, and sometimes on an assertion that the state's interest in preserving life diminishes in the face of an inexorable dying process.[30] In the ground-breaking *Quinlan* case, the court commented:

> We would see . . . a real distinction between the self-infliction of deadly harm and a self-determination against artificial life support or radical surgery, for instance, in the face of irreversible, painful and certain imminent death.[31]

In short, both popular perception and judicial doctrine regard the self-determination of an irreversibly terminally ill patient as exempt from moral and legal condemnations of suicide. The public policy which discourages suicide is simply not applied to a stricken patient who chooses not to delay an inevitable and approaching demise. The judicial technique, as noted, is to rely on absence of specific intent to die or absence of a self-initiated action in order to distinguish between suicide and rejection of life-preserving medical treatment by a dying patient.

For patients facing death from non self-induced trauma, but who are potentially salvageable to a lengthy and "healthful" existence, the relationship between their resistance to life-preserving treatment and suicide is more murky. In such situations, the patient is seeking to assert interests in medical self-determination and freedom from unwanted bodily invasion, but the element of an inexorable dying process is absent.

There are some courts and commentators who insist that in the absence of an irresistable disease, a patient's rejection of treatment is tantamount to suicide and warrants judicial intervention to override the patient's decision. This was the result in at least two instances when courts ordered blood transfusions for young accident victims who were salvageable to healthful existences.[32] In one of those cases, Judge J. Skelly Wright, an eminent jurist, specifically analogized the patient's refusal of treatment to suicide. He commented:

> [W]here attempted suicide is illegal by common law or by statute, a person may not be allowed to refuse necessary medical assistance when death is likely to ensue without it. Only quibbles about the distinction between misfeasance and nonfeasance [action or inaction], or the specific intent necessary to be guilty of attempted suicide, could be raised against this latter conclusion.[33]

Despite Judge Wright's assertion, the bulk of legal authority is to the contrary. In the context of salvageable patients making principled, religiously grounded decisions to resist life-preserving treatment, the majority of courts are now willing to acquiesce in the patient's exercise of self-determination and bodily control (at least in the absence of a further state interest such as protection of the patient's minor children).

The spectre of suicide can be averted by relying on Judge Wright's "quibble" that the religiously motivated patient has no specific intent to die. (In fact, such a patient wants desperately to live, but fears eternal damnation by acceptance of a blood transfusion.) Moreover, the distinction regarding specific intent is more than a quibble. Though the religiously motivated patient may die for a reason which appears silly or inconsequential to many observers, neither the patient's decision nor the court's acquiescence disparages the reverence for life which in part underlies antisuicide laws. The patient's determination to reject life-saving treatment reflects a principled invocation of personal and religious convictions, not a deprecation of life. Judicial restraint is impelled by profound respect for the individual's bodily integrity and religious freedom, not by disregard or disdain for the sanctity of life.

Antisuicide laws have never meant that life is the supreme value in American society. Such laws have always coexisted with capital punishment and authority to wage wars, for example. It comes as no shock, then, that courts now refuse to apply antisuicide predilections to religiously motivated refusals of life-saving medical treatment. Additionally, the "illegality" of attempted suicide, upon which Judge Wright grounded his 1966 analysis, no longer represents the current state of the law. Attempted suicide is no longer deemed a criminal offense.

As noted in chapter 1, a small number of courts have gone further, and acquiesced in rejections of life-saving treatment by salvageable patients who invoked not religious principles, but personal distaste for the dismal nature of the salvageable existence at hand. These cases dealt primarily with elderly patients spurning amputations to arrest gangrene, or with the continuation of dialysis treatment to combat chronic kidney disease. In these contexts, the potential tension with antisuicide policies is stronger, for the specific intention of the patient may be to die. This is so where the patient's condition is dismal before the proposed medical intervention as well as afterward—as with the dialysis patient who can't stand the dependency and intrusiveness of twelve hours a week on the machine.

The practical explanation for judicial willingness to circumvent antisuicide predispositions in this context is empathy for the patient's resistance to the prospect of a debilitated existence. Judges, being people, can understand a previously vigorous patient's antipathy to life as an amputee. Hence a willingness exists to endorse what might appear to many, including the judges themselves, as a "foolish" decision to resist life-preserving therapy. But there is a sound theoretical basis as well for differentiating these rejections of treatment from suicide. A medical patient facing a potentially fatal disease and resisting therapy is exercising a widely recognized prerogative to determine which medical interventions will be tolerated.

This patient prerogative is operative from the simplest decision whether to take an aspirin on up to whether to undergo a heart transplant operation. The reported cases tend to emphasize the extent of the bodily invasion entailed—such as in an amputation operation—but I have argued that the interest in patient autonomy should prevail even where the bodily invasion is less pronounced. For a patient whose existence has become a subjectively intolerable burden (perhaps because of the spectre of an inevitable gradual loss of faculties awaiting a victim of Alzheimer's disease), a decision to terminate simplistic procedures such as antibiotics or nutrition ought to be an option. This is part of the medical patient's prerogative to individually assess the merits and demerits of the proposed medical interventions.

Hunger Strikes and Starvation as Rejection of Medical Therapy

Where a patient has self-induced a terminal condition, as where a previously healthy person undertakes to starve to death, the tension between refusal of life-preserving therapy and traditional public aversion to suicide is intense. While rejection of nutrition does constitute a passive resistance to a bodily invasion, the fact that the mortal threat stems from a self-generated as opposed to a natural trauma smacks mightily of suicide. One commentator has observed:

> The 'passive' refusal of food in the depressed person or in the hunger striker is every bit as much a cause of death over which the person has control as is the proverbial bottle of barbiturates.[34]

Not surprisingly, then, the courts, primarily in the context of prisoners engaged in hunger strikes, have tended to reject the analogy of a starving person to a terminally ill medical patient refusing treatment. They have tended to authorize forced feeding. In the prison context, government intervention is reinforced by a reluctance to allow institutionalized persons to manipulate administrators through the hunger strike tactic. But in the noted *Bouvia* case[35], as well, the California court was persuaded that the paraplegic patient's plea to be allowed to starve to death was tantamount to suicide and warranted state intervention at least so long as Ms. Bouvia chose to remain in a government hospital.

I can't fault the legal analysis in this line of cases in which the patient's terminal condition results from an entirely self-induced etiology. The refusal of nutrition in such an instance is indeed *tantamount* to suicide. Nevertheless, I would suggest that nonprisoners, such as Elizabeth Bouvia, and prisoners who are not seeking to extract promises from their jailors, ought to be permitted to starve to death if that is their considered wish. This position flows from a strong sympathy for individual self-determination, along with a conviction that at least some of the normal state interests in suicide prevention are not really at stake.

The principal objective of governmental intervention in the area of suicide is to secure assistance for the troubled individual. Such assistance is appropriate because many suicide attempts are the product of rash, unbalanced, or confused judgments. While there is no simple explanation for the phenomenon of suicide, and reference is frequently made to a "profound ambiguity of motives," some suicide attempts are the product of mental disorder. Some attempts are acknowledged to be either conscious or unconscious cries for help, rather than determined efforts to die. No criticism can be directed toward governmental efforts to reach and assist persons who do not wish to die or whose suicidal action is the product of a temporary derangement. "The natural and human thing to do with a person who is suddenly discovered attempting suicide is to interpose to prevent it."[36]

If a person is competent and reaches a firm and deliberate determination to starve to death, the state interest in preventing rash or unbalanced self-destruction is not implicated. So long as there are no dependents who would be grievously harmed by the person's decision, and so long as the requisite mental competence is present, the decision to reject nutrition should be respected. The incidence of such "suicides" is not likely to be great. There are much quicker and efficient means to accomplish the task if a person is determined to die. Elizabeth Bouvia presented a rare situation where the person's physical handicaps prevented other means of self-destruction.

Another consideration is that the means necessary to overcome the will of a person resisting feeding are repulsive. A person determined to resist an intravenous tube would normally have to be restrained physically or doped up regularly during periods of nutrition administration. For a society that normally respects both bodily integrity and individual autonomy, the spectre of forced feeding is indeed repulsive. I personally would prefer to respect a person's determination—reiterated over the period during which starvation would last—that their life is too painful to endure.

Both physical and emotional pain are intensely subjective notions. When a person like Elizabeth Bouvia makes an initial judgment that her debilitated existence is too painful to be worth preserving, counseling should be provided in order to outline all perspectives and to seek to dissuade the patient. If she persists in her considered wish to resist nutrition, and if medical personnel are available who are willing in good conscience to provide the palliative care which she seeks during the dying process, I think that her decision should be respected. Obviously, I am willing to allow quality of life determinations to enter the medical context, a proposition that deserves attention because it suffuses the whole debate over death and dying, and raises hackles in many medical and legal sources.

Quality of Life in Terminal Decisions

In some circles, the mention of quality of life as a relevant factor in death and dying decision-making evokes strenuous objections. The concern is that any acknowledgement that a life is "not worth living" opens the way for injecting factors into terminal decisions that will be subject to grave abuse. For example, some commentators argue that utilitarian concerns such as the economic burden of keeping certain persons alive will corrupt the decision-making process and undermine society's traditional respect for the value of life. They fear a substitution of a "quality of life" ethic for a "sanctity of life" ethic with an attendant injection of a "cost-benefit morality" in the approach to terminal decisions.[37]

The implication is that the poor or helpless would be victimized under such criteria. Once quality of life is viewed as an acceptable concept, it is argued, there are a wide variety of populations who might be deemed too great a burden for society, or better off dead than alive. These include the handicapped, insane, retarded, senile, sickly, incorrigibly poor, or unwanted. We are frequently reminded that the Nazi holocaust was signalled by incredible inhumanity toward the sick and defective under the justification that their lives were not worth preserving, or that their lives were dispensable for the greater social good.

These concerns must be taken quite seriously. Quality of life, as used by some sources, does carry with it some connotation of "worthiness" or social utility which is alarming, particularly in the context of incompetent patients. This spectre is occasionally discernible in the context of defective newborns. There, some discussions seem to consider whether an infant's existence is worth preserving, not from the perspective of pain and suffering to be incurred by the handicapped child, but from concern about deviance from normalcy. There is a tendency to equate a significantly impaired existence with an unacceptable quality of life— that is, an assumption is made that life without full faculties is disposable at infancy either because the interests of parents and society to be free of burdens are more weighty, or because a being cannot really enjoy a significantly impaired existence.

Yet the fact that people sometimes distort a principle does not mean that the principle must be discarded rather than refined. Any salutary principle is subject to abuse, and it is important to carefully define and analyze the principle in order to determine whether it can be confined to its appropriate bounds. That approach must be undertaken with regard to quality of life as a factor in terminal decisions.

In the context of a competent person deciding what medical treatment to undergo, quality of life by no means imports social utility or "worthiness" factors. The reality is that every medical decision is suffused with quality of life judgments. In deciding whether to take an aspirin, a person principally considers quality of life—the discomfort experienced without medication versus the degree of relief likely with the pill. In addition, the person might consider any possible side effects (from allergies or whatever), and possibly the expense entailed.

Such everyday medical decisions don't normally implicate death as a consideration. But sometimes, a choice of therapy, with its attendant weighing of quality of life factors, entails mortal risks. This was vividly illustrated not long ago in the case of the "bubble boy." There, a youth with an immune deficiency was removed from his safe and sterile, but terribly confining, "plastic bubble" environment in an effort to use a therapy which would permit freedom of movement. The experiment failed and the youth died. But no one blamed the youth or his family for taking a mortal risk in order to improve the quality of his existence from extraordinarily confined to normal. (Although the youth was a minor, I assume that he had a large role in the familial decision. In any event, the legal and moral conclusions would not have changed if the bubble boy had been a twenty-one-year-old adult. The determination to risk death in order to achieve a better quality of life would still have been respected.)[38]

The key factor with competent patients is that an autonomous person is making a judgment about what course of medical treatment to undertake according to his or her own assessment of advantages and disadvantages. Inevitably, the quality of the existence available with or without the therapy is a consideration. In the context of the terminally ill, the patient typically considers the prospect of physical pain as a major factor. But there are a variety of subjective emotional pains which come into play—dependence, helplessness, and loss of dignity—any or all of which may play a prominent role in an ultimate decision, and all of which are quality of life factors.

Nor is a person facing a potentially terminal condition confined to consideration of his or her own current and prospective status. The emotional strain and financial burden posed to loved ones may play a significant role in the dying patient's decision when to resist efforts to prolong the dying process. To phrase it differently, embarrassment at posing a burden to others may be part of the emotional suffering which a competent patient considers when deciding whether to accept life-preserving medical intervention.

Most people die from chronic deteriorations associated with aging. Some persons determine at some point in the process that diminished and disordered function is no longer bearable. I suggest that at that point they may choose to resist medical intervention accompanying any potentially fatal illness.

What distinguishes the decision to refuse life-sustaining care from other medical decisions is the implicit judgment that death is more desirable to the patient than the level of existence salvageable. Some commentators have a very hard time acknowledging that life can become so burdensome as to be relinquishable. Such a life-repudiating judgment is offensive to those who view life as *the* supreme good, to be preserved at all cost. Nonetheless, most people appear to accept what the courts have tended to endorse—that at least where a patient is confronting an inexorable dying process, the patient is entitled to determine when the actual or prospective existence has become so "painful" as to prompt a rejection of life-sustaining care. Thus, the terminally ill cancer patient has a prerogative to determine whether to undergo the strains of chemotherapy. And the patient facing chronic degenerative diseases leading to massive incapacity and death—such as Alzheimer's disease or Lou Gehrig's disease—ought to be able to pick the point at which debilitation is no longer tolerable. A recent *New York Times* article reports that "negotiated deaths" are becoming a common phenomenon in cases of this type.[39] In such arrangements, an intermediary such as an attorney undertakes obtaining understandings from medical and prosecutorial officials that they will not intervene in the removal of life-sustaining equipment pursuant to the patient's request.

There is nothing alarming or distasteful in such deference to patient judgments about quality of life. What is sad is that the emerging consensus to respect patient self-determination is not universally recognized. It is sad that medical institutions still occasionally resist a competent, dying patient's determination to decline medical intervention and that they then force the patient to undertake expensive and emotionally wrenching litigation.

In the recent *Bartling* incident in California, doctors refused to remove a respirator at the request of a seventy-year-old patient suffering from five normally fatal diseases including cancer and emphysema.[40] Part of the explanation offered was that death was not sufficiently "imminent." This seems to me to be a misguided concern. I have already argued that the terminally ill patient deserves a prerogative to fix the point at which existence is so "painful" that resistance may cease. That prerogative ought not be confined to the brief span when death is "imminent." To rule otherwise is to diminish patient autonomy and to condemn patients to subjective suffering up until that point of imminence. Humane medical practice does not require such a result; respect for patient self-determination dictates a contrary result.

There is a quality of life judgment being made by the resisting patient whether death is imminent or not—the determination is that an earlier death is preferable to lingering in a debilitated and painful state during the inexorable dying process. In the case of "imminence," the quality of life determination is simply a shorter term decision.

The courts have begun to accept the competent, terminally ill patient's prerogative to shape the dying process. The problem now is to reach a level of medical and public consciousness at which there will be no need to litigate in order to implement what should be understood as the terminally ill patient's prerogative.

Quality of life is a much more problematical element in the context of incompetent persons. There patient autonomy may not occupy the prominent role it does for competent patients. I will turn in chapter 3 to the whole subject of handling incompetent patients. Suffice it to say for now that "quality of life," properly defined, is an important factor even in that context. As a practical matter, hundreds or even thousands of quality of life judgments confront medical personnel and patient guardians daily in dealing with terminally ill patients who have lost the mental capacity to make their own choices of treatment. The duration and quality of remaining existence (quality from the perspective of the patient) is inevitably a principal criterion in deciding whether to initiate life-preserving machinery, whether to withdraw it once instituted, and whether to resuscitate in the event of cardiopulmonary failure. Such considerations cannot be averted in the medical arena.

Official recognition and sanction of this fact have come in several different forms. Perhaps the earliest endorsement of quality of life judgments came in gradual acceptance of brain death, rather than respiratory failure, as an official mark of death. While it may be possible to mechanically sustain breathing and blood circulation in a brain dead being for some time, that being can experience no pleasure or pain or social interaction whatsoever. Hence the unobjectionable conclusion that the quality of existence is so low that machinery may be removed and the remains buried.

A similar quality of life assessment might prevail in the case of permanent coma. In the reknowned *Quinlan* case, the New Jersey Supreme Court in effect endorsed a guardian's quality of life determination that a person in a permanently comatose state (though not brain dead) might legally and humanely be allowed to expire via removal of a respirator. The patient herself was presumably experiencing no pain or discomfort in her lingering state. But her status was so dismal that preservation constituted no gain or benefit to her; that marginal existence need not be preserved, ruled the court.

As will be seen in more detail in the pages immediately following, duration and quality of existence have also become an accepted criteria with regard to terminally ill incompetent patients who are not comatose. Because such patients are by definition helpless to assert their own interests, and because their continued existence may be financially and emotionally draining on those persons around them, there is a hazard that unsavory utilitarian factors may enter the calculus of when to withhold life-preserving care. For that reason, quality of life must be carefully defined according to the perspectives of the patient—either as expressed previous to becoming incompetent, or as gleaned from common understanding of a person's best interests.[41] In pursuit of that object, I turn to the question of what criteria govern decisions on behalf of incompetent, terminally ill patients.

III

HANDLING INCOMPETENT PATIENTS:
Decision-Making Criteria

To this point, discussion has centered on the prerogative of medical patients to shape their own dying process by deciding which medical interventions to accept. Yet, multitudes of patients lack sufficient mental understanding of their condition, treatment options, and consequences to be considered legally competent to make such decisions for themselves. For many patients, this period of incompetence is the culmination of a gradual deterioration during a protracted dying process. Faculties and capacities may simply weaken as death approaches, with the patient ultimately lapsing into a comatose or semi-comatose state. Death may then occur either in an acute care hospital or in a long-term care facility, such as a nursing home.

For other patients, incompetence has been a characteristic long before the onset of some fatal condition. These may be adults who suffer severe senile dementia over a protracted period. Still other patients have never been competent. These may be people who have been severely retarded from birth or a childhood trauma. Many in this latter population languish in public institutions for the mentally handicapped. There, critical medical decisions arise not just in the context of lethal illnesses such as cancer, but when potentially fatal conditions such as pneumonia or heart attack arise. Or a patient may be so impaired that artificial feeding—through a surgically implanted tube, for example—is a part of their ongoing existence.

For all of these patients, life and death decisions must be made by someone on their behalf. Numerous questions inevitably arise. Who is authorized to make a terminal decision regarding an incompetent patient? What processes of consultation or approval must be followed? And, most importantly, what criteria or standards govern a decision to withhold or withdraw life-preserving care from an incompetent, dying patient? This chapter addresses the problem of criteria for decision-making; the questions of who decides, and with what kinds of consultation, will be considered in chapter 5.

The New Jersey Supreme Court has been a leading force in this area through major decisions in 1976 and 1985. The ground-breaking efforts by the New Jersey court can serve as a useful introduction to a discussion of decision-making criteria for incompetent, dying patients. For those rulings will have a marked influence on how other states resolve the legal issues surrounding the withdrawal of life-preserving care from incompetent patients.

In re Quinlan,[1] decided in 1976, was the first major judicial decision establishing that life-supporting medical procedures may, in certain circumstances, be withdrawn from a dying patient lacking the mental capacity to make his own medical choices. Karen Ann Quinlan was a twenty-two-year-old woman who, after ingesting a mixture of alcohol and drugs, lapsed into a permanent and irreversible coma. Ms. Quinlan was not dead by any legal standard, as her brain stem continued to function and to regulate body temperature, breathing, heart rate, swallowing, blinking, and reaction to noxious stimuli. But Ms. Quinlan had no chance of returning to consciousness, to a cognitive existence, and her family wished to discontinue a respirator that was thought to be sustaining her tenuous life. When treating physicians hesitated to disconnect the respirator, her father sought judicial approval to act as a legal guardian and to have the respirator discontinued.

In a unanimous decision, the New Jersey Supreme Court effectively removed the prior fear that removal or withholding of a life-support system from an incompetent patient would inevitably be treated as homicide and/or medical malpractice. The *Quinlan* court ruled that a terminal decision might be made by a natural guardian, such as a next of kin, with concurrence by the treating physician, the family, and the medical institution's "ethics committee."[2]

The permissible circumstances, or general standards to guide decision-makers, were more murky. The guide for permanently comatose patients such as Ms. Quinlan was clearly provided. Her respirator could be removed upon finding "no reasonable possibility of Karen's ever emerging from her present comatose condition to a cognitive, sapient state. . . ."[3] But there were a variety of hints about standards to guide future terminal decisions not involving permanently comatose patients.

Some reliance was placed in *Quinlan* on a patient's decision to reject treatment as a fundamental aspect of personal privacy safeguarded against state intrusion by the fourteenth amendment to the federal Constitution. The guardian would then be implementing the patient's own constitutional prerogative to resist life-preserving treatment. Consistent with this approach, the opinion instructed Ms. Quinlan's guardians to "render their best judgment" as to whether she would have exercised her right to resist treatment if she had been somehow able to decide for herself in the situation confronting her. Yet the court also, surprisingly, disavowed any reliance on Ms. Quinlan's previous comments to her family about being sustained in a comatose state; those expressions were regarded as too remote in time and too casual.[4]

Other language in *Quinlan* provided some basis for applying other decision-making formulas. For example, the court expressed an intention to promote medical practices conducted "for the well being of . . . dying patients." This language would support a standard geared to the "best interests" of the incompetent, moribund patient. At the same time, the court endorsed relief from the dying process where continued medical intervention offers "neither human nor humane benefit." Relief from the irremediable limbo of insensate coma was in effect deemed "humane."[5]

Quinlan also did not fully resolve what kinds of medical procedures can be withdrawn or withheld. The court authorized removal of a respirator. But Ms. Quinlan survived when the respirator was removed. The court did not consider whether more basic medical support, such as administration of antibiotics or artificial nourishment, could be terminated.[6]

In January 1985, in a case called *In re Conroy*,[7] the New Jersey Supreme Court provided further guidance both as to standards of decision-making for incompetent patients and types of medical support potentially removable from a dying patient. In *Conroy*, the court addressed the thorny issue of elderly, incompetent patients suffering from chronic, degenerative conditions whose lives have reached their last stages, but who are not facing immediately life-threatening conditions.

Claire Conroy was an eighty-four-year-old nursing home resident afflicted with severe organic brain syndrome (senility), along with urinary tract infection, a gangrenous leg, arteriosclerotic heart disease, hypertension, and diabetes mellitus. She was bedridden and unable to move from a semi-fetal position. She was not comatose, but her intellectual capacity was extremely limited. She was severely demented and unable to respond to verbal stimuli. She could not speak. In response to physical stimuli, Ms. Conroy exhibited minor movement of the hands or head. Medical testimony was "inconclusive" about her ability to experience pain. She would make occasional moaning sounds, would occasionally pull at her bandages or tubes, and would occasionally smile in response to stroking. She was incontinent. In the course of her decline,

Ms. Conroy had lost the ability to swallow and a naso-gastric feeding tube had been installed two years earlier. At the time her case came to court in 1983, Ms. Conroy lay immobile and virtually insensate, staring ahead, sustained by nutrients passed through her feeding tube.

In 1983, Ms. Conroy's sole relative, a nephew, sought judicial authorization to have her naso-gastric tube removed so that she could be allowed to die. Upon removal of the tube, Ms. Conroy would die from dehydration in about a week. Otherwise, the medical projection was that she could languish for a few months or longer.

The trial court was willing to grant the nephew's petition. The lower court judge ruled that where intellectual function has been permanently reduced to such a primitive level and life with an array of medical afflictions has become "impossibly burdensome," artificial nourishment can be withdrawn and the patient permitted to die. This could be done even though, according to one doctor's testimony, the demise through starvation might be "painful."[8]

The intermediate appellate court refused to go along with this approach.[9] That court ruled that routine life support, such as nutrition, could not be withdrawn from a patient who was neither permanently comatose nor in a terminal condition in which death was irreversibly imminent. The appellate court did not dispute the nephew's contention that Ms. Conroy, if competent, would have wanted to be withdrawn from the artificial nutrition. But the court found no strong indication that she was suffering in her debilitated state, while there was some indication that death by starvation might be painful.

The New Jersey Supreme Court reversed the decision. That court ruled that a naso-gastric tube is a form of "artificial feeding" classifiable as a medical procedure and potentially withdrawable from a dying medical patient. In the case of incompetent nursing home residents suffering from "severe and permanent mental and physical impairments" who will die within one year even with full treatment, the court fixed both the process and the criteria for making a decision to withdraw artificial feeding or other life-preserving medical treatment.[10]

The process outlined by the Court was somewhat complex. Before any terminal decision can be made regarding an incompetent nursing home resident, there must be a judicial finding supported by at least two examining physicians that the patient himself lacks competence to make treatment determinations. Then, the initial determination to remove or withhold life-sustaining treatment can be made by a guardian, so long as the guardian has been appointed by a court which has examined the guardian's qualifications and good faith. But before implementation, the guardian's terminal decision must gain concurrence from several sources. First, the medical prognosis has to be verified by two physicians independent of the nursing home. Then, the decision itself has to be supported by an attending physician, by the patient's close family, and by an investigating "ombudsman"—a New Jersey public employee (from the Department of Community Affairs) normally charged with safeguarding the interests of institutionalized individuals. All of these sources will scrutinize the guardian's determination. In the event that one of these sources fails to concur in a terminal decision, the guardian would presumably have to secure judicial approval if he wished to proceed with the initial determination.[11]

As to decision-making criteria, the court first formulated what it deemed a "subjective test." Under that test, the initial objective is to determine the subjective wishes of the now incompetent patient. This starting point—a search for the now incompetent patient's preferences—is consistent with the New Jersey court's position that every person enjoys a common law right to determine what medical interventions will be performed on himself. As in the case of a constitutional right of privacy, the common law right to medical self-determination subsists after the patient becomes incompetent, so long as the patient's previous competently expressed wishes can be discerned.

The incompetent patient's wishes must be gleaned by examining prior expressions (living will, oral declaration, etc.) or less direct evidence of the patient's preferences and tastes. (This willingness to consider prior statements from the patient constituted a reversal of the bar previously imposed in the *Quinlan* case.) Where the patient's competently expressed wishes can be ascertained, the court indicated that they should be implemented by the surrogate decision-maker. Where the specific wishes of the patient are not discernible, the court articulated a standard—to be discussed in detail below—which can roughly be characterized as "best interests of the patient." The object then becomes to decide whether the burdens or hardships of a patient's prospective existence with treatment outweigh the prospective benefits of the preservable life.

Since Ms. Conroy had never given a clear indication of her wishes regarding terminal treatment, the court indicated that the best interests test was applicable. Yet the *Conroy* court did not resolve whether the nephew's decision to seek removal of his aunt's naso-gastric tube was appropriate according to the best interests standard. The issue was moot in any event because Ms. Conroy had died while the litigation was pending. Nonetheless, the indeterminative result was not grounded on mootness. Rather, the judges all felt that the record was too bare to definitively decide whether Ms. Conroy's best interests would have been served by removal of the feeding tube. Sufficient data was lacking concerning Ms. Conroy's prior expressions and value systems, as well as medical information concerning the nature of pain currently plaguing the patient or likely to accompany a starvation process.

The bottom line of both *Quinlan* and *Conroy* is that there are circumstances in which life-preserving medical care may legally be withheld from an incompetent patient. The two decisions, taken in conjunction, also suggest that there are a variety of possible formulations to describe the standard or guideline for a surrogate decision-maker. In this chapter, I will examine the merits of the two principal standards which emerge from these two decisions (as well as from the cases decided in other jurisdictions)—namely, the "subjective" or "substituted judgment" standard and the "best interests" standard. I'll then offer an alternative analysis which goes beyond the best interests approach ultimately endorsed by *Conroy*. Finally, at the end of this chapter I'll address some of the pending questions which neither the substituted judgment nor best interests formula really resolves.

Substituted Judgment

Whether a patient's prerogative to spurn life-preserving treatment is grounded on constitutional privacy or on the common law doctrine of informed consent, the object remains to honor individual dignity by promoting self-determination and choice. In the context of a previously competent patient who has become incompetent, that object is accomplished most clearly by implementing the wishes of the patient as expressed at a point when the patient was competent. The term "substituted judgment" is commonly used to describe this approach in which the subjective intent of the formerly competent patient is allowed to govern.

Under the substituted judgment approach, the surrogate decision-maker must effectuate, to the extent possible, the course of conduct which the patient would have desired. "The decision should be that which would be made by the incompetent person, if he were competent, taking into account his actual interests and preferences. . . ."[12] This was essentially the tack taken by the *Conroy* court in formulating what it termed its "subjective test." The court observed: "[T]he goal of decision-making for incompetent patients should be to determine and effectuate, insofar as possible, the decision that the patient would have made if competent."[13] This approach—seeking to discover and implement what the particular patient would have done if able to choose for himself—has been endorsed by a number of other courts, as well.

Since genuine self-determination entails considered weighing of alternative courses of action, the best device in this context would be a prior directive in which the patient addresses the situations in which the patient would prefer that medical intervention cease. In other words, the best way to implement patient autonomy in the death and dying context is by considering a patient's prior expressions regarding circumstances in which death would be preferred over continued existence.

As to such prior expressions of intent, the *Conroy* court commented that probative value "may vary depending on the remoteness, consistency, and thoughtfulness of the prior statements or actions and the maturity of the person at the time of the statements or acts."[14] But the prior expressions are at least to be considered by surrogate decision-makers "for what they are worth." According to the *Conroy* court, less direct evidence of intent may also be examined. This might include such elements as the patient's religious beliefs, or a consistent pattern of conduct regarding prior medical treatment. Life-preserving treatment may be withheld where it is clear from the patient's prior statements and conduct that the patient would have refused such treatment under the circumstances involved.

There are limits to the utility of the substituted judgment approach. Even when a person takes the unusual step of contemplating future incapacity and making an advance directive, implementation may prove problematical. The wide variety of potential illnesses, prognoses, conditions, and treatments may result in vague directions which are not much practical help when the time comes for implementation. Moreover, a person's views are subject to change with time and new perspectives. As one physician has observed:

> [P]ersons' ideas about the quality of life change drastically as they age, especially in the last years of their lives. The twenty-one-year-old who wants to be shot rather than suffer the imagined ignominy of a nursing home is only too grateful to accept the nursing home bed and warm meals when he turns eighty-five. A living will or a frank conversation with one's physician even at age fifty-five would rarely reflect what one's wishes would be at seventy.[15]

These understandable problems with remoteness and abstractness of expression may impede a guardian's effort to effectuate previous directions. The *Conroy* court's anticipation that the probative value of declarations will vary according to their proximity and specificity is surely correct. Nonetheless, respect for patient autonomy requires that every effort be made to discern and fulfill the patient's own preferences as previously communicated.

The substituted judgment approach correctly seeks to implement a competent person's right of self-determination, to the extent feasible, even after the patient has lost competence to make further determinations. This implementation of prior decisions is enormously important. Some incompetent patients may actually feel and appreciate the effectuation of their value choices. That is, some languishing patients, though not sufficiently aware to make a competent medical decision, may have enough awareness to sense and appreciate relief when painful, intrusive, or embarrassing care is withdrawn in accordance with the patient's prior instructions. Moreover, even if the patient is too insensate to appreciate the honoring of his or her choice, effectuation of that choice is important. American society values human dignity, and an essential component of that human dignity is the making of intimate decisions according to personal priorities and preferences.[16] Traditionally, that decision-making authority has extended even to matters which will take effect only after a person's death. Thus, American law allows a person to determine the postmortem fate of his or her organs—their availability or unavailability for transplantation, and, laws of testamentary disposition allow a competent person to determine how his property will be allocated after his death. These approaches honoring self-determination are obviously salutary even though the decision-maker will be insensate at the moment when the decisions are implemented.

Citizens benefit from the knowledge that their wishes concerning the dying process will be respected even after they have lost awareness of the consequences. People care now about the prospect of future maintenance in a debilitated, helpless state even though they may not fully sense degradation when the incompetent state is reached. Just as part of the value of privacy is peace of mind from knowing that one will not be covertly intruded upon, a benefit extends to people by knowing that their dying process will not be needlessly prolonged. Whether their concern is to avoid suffering, or to avoid crippling expenses to their estate, or simply not to be remembered in a deteriorated condition, people can appreciate the assurance that their wishes will be honored. Any other approach would permit obliteration of a competent person's decisions at any point at which the person subsequently becomes incompetent. A competent patient's shaping of the dying process could then be ignored as soon as the patient deteriorated. Such a result would badly undermine patient autonomy in the death and dying context.

Sometimes, previous directives will provide firm guidance in the handling of a terminally ill, incompetent patient. For example, in one recent case, a comatose patient had conducted long and careful discussions with a colleague in which the patient expressed the wish, repeated within months of falling into a coma, not to be maintained in a permanently comatose state. The patient's wish was respected there, just as it was in another instance where a now comatose patient had previously expressed a wish not to be maintained in a "vegetative state."[17]

In the many instances when an incompetent patient never articulates preferences about the dying process and limits of intolerable living conditions, some sources urge careful assessment of the patient's character, tastes, and previous patterns of behavior in order to exercise substituted judgment and decide how the patient would want to be handled.[18] On occasion, that inquiry can be fruitful. For example, the patient's firmly held religious beliefs may dictate that a particular course of treatment not be followed. On other occasions, guardians and judges have used fairly oblique evidence of a patient's character to conclude that the patient would want life-preserving treatment discontinued. Examples of this phenomenon are not hard to find. In *In re Colyer*,[19] a husband relied on his wife's independent nature and dislike of physicians to project that she would not wish to be preserved in a brain-damaged, persistently vegetative state. A similar decision was reached by a court in *In re Torres*,[20] grounded in part on testimony that the now comatose patient had been a vigorous person who had resisted wearing a heart pacemaker. General lifestyle of the formerly competent patient was also used in part in *In re Spring*[21] to support a determination by a wife and son that the senile, seventy-eight-year-old husband and father would want to be removed from kidney dialysis treatment despite a prognosis that the patient could live up to five more years with continued treatment.

Substantial criticism has been voiced about such efforts to apply a substituted judgment analysis in the absence of a patient's prior considered expressions about terminal care, or a well-developed philosophical or religious position. One contention is that a decision-maker, in drawing from a patient's lifetime of behavior and experience, can focus on elements most consistent with the decision-maker's own preconceptions and views about the handling of incompetent patients. The suggestion is that substituted judgment can become a charade, and that it would be better to direct the decision-maker to assess the best interests of the incompetent patient rather than to conduct an abortive search for what the patient would have done for himself.[22]

While substituted judgment may be a problematical standard for a guardian to administer, it cannot be dispensed with altogether. Even though people are normally presumed to act in their own best interests, so that there will inevitably be some overlap between what the patient allegedly would have done and the patient's best interests, substituted judgment must remain the starting point for any guardian's decision-making process. For there will be situations in which the patient's wishes should be followed, even though they dictate a decision contrary to the patient's best interests as measured in traditional terms of benefit to the incompetent patient's own interests and well being.

A few examples may help illustrate situations where the patient's subjective wishes will deviate from what are normally considered best interests of the patient. The incompetent patient may have been a person with great solicitude toward his family. He or she might well have expressed a desire to have terminal care decisions made with a view toward the economic and emotional burdens imposed on the surrounding family members during the patient's dying process. While these burdens on persons other than the patient are not normally considered part of the patient's best interests, a patient's altruism may be an acceptable part of the personal values implemented through the substituted judgment focus on self-determination. Similarly, implementation of a patient's aberrational or unusual wishes fits more comfortably within the rubric of substituted judgment than best interests. This applies to the patient whose religious scruples dictate refusal of a blood transfusion, or to the patient whose aversion to physical incapacity dictates refusal of a life-preserving amputation. A patient's guardian or surrogate decision-maker ought to be able to reject treatment in the same circumstances in which the patient, if competent, could exercise that prerogative. The self-determination and autonomy underlying substituted judgment provide the rationale for allowing the guardian to follow the patient's aberrational wishes, so long as those wishes have been clearly communicated.

The recent President's Commission has taken a somewhat contrary position. That group claims that certain decisions "adverse" to the interests of the incompetent patient are beyond the realm of a surrogate decision-maker's authority.[23] Use of experimental medical procedures is given as an illustration. That position, however, contravenes the principle of self-determination on which substituted judgment is based. Patient autonomy includes idiosyncratic wishes even though they might not seem wise or prudent to most people—subject always to the caveat that the patient's intentions are clearly expressed. Thus, if a competent person dictates that he wishes to participate in a nontherapeutic experimental medical procedure, I see no bar to implementing that instruction even after the patient has become incompetent, and even though observers might feel that the experimental medical procedure is not in the patient's best interests.

Best Interests of the Incompetent Patient

Many dying persons never provide intelligible instructions concerning their medical handling. Some patients are victims of sudden and traumatic injury or illness and reach an incompetent stage without ever having given considered expression to their desires concerning death. The vast majority of people simply prefer not to relate to the macabre subject of death and dying unless it is thrust upon them. Even some dying persons faced with gradual degeneration may refuse to acknowledge their condition before they have deteriorated to a point of incompetency. Some people have been incompetent since birth and never possessed the capacity to make medical decisions.

The *Conroy* decision recognized both that actual patient preferences will be undiscernible in many instances, and that "in the absence of adequate proof of the patient's wishes, it is naive to pretend that the right to self-determination serves as the basis for substituted decision-making."[24] The point is well taken. Self-determination normally requires an individualized assertion of tastes, preferences, and priorities on the part of a competent being. Usually this means an exercise of choice contemporaneous with the medical circumstances facing the patient. Free choice may also be meaningful when an individual's prior instructions are implemented after the individual has become incompetent. Where a patient has never articulated personal preferences about death, the dying process, and tolerable burdens in the face of death, it is somewhat presumptuous to purport to be effectuating patient choice.

In acknowledging these factors, *Conroy* averted a basic error, mentioned above, which had plagued predecessor courts. This was the attempt to articulate and apply a "substituted judgment" standard— deciding what the now incompetent patient would want done under the current circumstances—in the absence of clearcut or meaningful indications of patient feelings about death and dying. I described, for example, how some courts have tried to use an incompetent patient's prior aversion to doctors and hospitals as a basis for a substituted judgment that the patient would resist life-preserving medical treatment. This appears to be a questionable premise, at least where the prior aversion was not in the context of a potentially fatal medical condition.

While the *Conroy* court realized that substituted judgment was largely a pretense in the absence of meaningful prior expressions by a patient, the court wished to promote humane handling for languishing patients who had not clearly expressed their own preferences. That is, the judges did not wish to condemn to an indefinite lingering state a dying patient whose continued existence is torturous, or of no net benefit to the patient, but who had lacked the foresight or opportunity to supply prior instructions. The solution adopted by the *Conroy* court was a "best interests of the patient" standard involving assessment of net benefit or burden to the patient from the preservable existence.

The best interests standard was broken down into two strands—denominated the "limited objective" and "pure objective" tests. Under the limited objective test, there must be "some trustworthy evidence" that the incompetent patient, if competent, would refuse treatment under the circumstances currently being confronted. This evidence might entail prior expressions which indicated distaste for life in a debilitated state, but expressions too vague or casual to constitute clear proof of the patient's subjective wishes under the substituted judgment approach. With some such "trustworthy" evidence, the decision-maker can withdraw life-preserving treatment if clearly satisfied "that the burdens of the patient's continued life with the treatment outweigh the benefits of that life for him."[25] This was further defined by the court as meaning that the patient will suffer unavoidable pain and that the net pain and suffering[26] "markedly outweigh any physical pleasure, emotional enjoyment, or intellectual satisfaction that the patient may still be able to derive from life."[27]

The pure objective test of best interests is applicable in the absence of any meaningful indication of the patient's subjective wishes about terminal care. As in the case of the limited-objective test, treatment is withdrawable if the net burdens of the patient's life with treatment would "clearly and markedly outweigh the benefits that the patient derives from life." Moreover, there must be "recurring, unavoidable and severe pain" such that "the effect of administering life-sustaining treatment would be inhumane."[28] In short, the main distinction between the "limited" and "pure" objective test is the presence in the former case of some significant indication of the patient's preferences. The consequence then is that the weighing of burdens and benefits to determine the net best interests of the patient would be undertaken with cognizance of those individual patient preferences.

The *Conroy* focus on best interests is fully consistent with traditional guardianship principles prescribing that a guardian occupies a trust or fiduciary relationship toward an incompetent ward. This normally means that the guardian must act only in the best interests of the ward. Application of such a fiduciary standard fits with the state's parens patriae interest in safeguarding the well being of citizens unable to care for themselves. Traditionally, the best interests standard was applied to guardians' decisions in handling the property of incompetent wards. The standard is adaptable to the medical context as well—for example, in decisions as to whether an incompetent person should undergo an abortion or sterilization or receive a particular medical therapy when ill.

Conroy is by no means the first authority for application of a best interests standard in the context of a possible decision to terminate life-sustaining care for an incompetent, terminally ill adult. That is, other sources have conceded that a declining patient may be "better off dead than alive" when viewed from the perspective of that patient's own interests. The recent President's Commission endorsed use of the standard "a patient's well being" in two separate reports regarding medical decisions on behalf of incompetents.[29] And several courts have turned to the best interests standard in the context of proxy decision-making on behalf of incompetent dying patients.[30]

One novelty in the *Conroy* formulation is the injection of an element of the patient's subjective intent into the framework of best interests (via the "limited-objective" test). As noted, that test is conditioned on finding some evidence that the patient would have desired termination of terminal care under the circumstances. Yet best interests are normally viewed as involving an objective assessment of benefits and burdens to the patient, rather than a search for the patient's preferences.

The theoretical tension can be resolved if it is conceded that implementation of a person's values and preferences can form part of that person's best interests. That is, if best interests are equated with patient well being, and the definition of patient well being can be shaped by the personal values and standards of the patient, then it makes sense to assess the patient's preferences regarding acceptable living circumstances when deciding whether the patient's best interests dictate termination of treatment under the circumstances confronted.

This deference to the personal value systems of the patient—while more natural and convincing where the patient's subjective wishes can be definitively discerned—might serve a useful function, even under what would normally be a purely objective best interests formula. Attention to prior expressions and habits of the incompetent patient might serve as a vehicle for assessing the likely level of emotional suffering being undergone by the incompetent patient, or the level of deterioration or disability tolerable to the patient. For example, it makes sense to think that a person who has always been particularly vigorous and independent may well suffer from helplessness, frustration, and embarrassment from being sustained in a permanently incapacitated, helpless, and dependent state. In short, examination of a patient's prior lifestyle is relevant in assessing the incompetent patient's well being in his terminal state, even if it does not provide a firm basis for pretending that the patient is making a considered exercise of self-determination. Unfortunately, it's not perfectly clear that the *Conroy* court intended to include likely emotional suffering in its "best interests" of the patient formula.

There are some indications in *Conroy* that—without clear prior directions from the patient sufficient to satisfy the "subjective" (substituted judgment) test—unremitting physical pain is to be a sine qua non for any decision that termination of life-preserving care is in the best interests of the patient. In articulating its "limited-objective" standard for determining when the burdens of prospective existence outweigh the benefits, the court commented:

> [W]e mean that the patient is suffering, and will continue to suffer throughout the expected duration of his life, *unavoidable pain,* and that the net burdens [pain and suffering] . . . markedly outweigh any physical pleasure, emotional enjoyment, or intellectual satisfaction that the patient may still be able to derive from life.[31]

Under the pure objective test, applicable to the patient who has left no trustworthy indication of his desires, "recurring, unavoidable and severe pain" was specified as a prerequisite to termination. The question is whether the pain referred to in either or both of these formulations is confined to physical rather than emotional pain.

It is unclear whether the *Conroy* majority really intended to make physical pain a sine qua non in this context. Certainly, the New Jersey Supreme Court was well aware that debilitated, waning patients sometimes suffer a variety of emotional insults. Under the subjective test aimed at implementing the wishes of the particular patient, the decision-maker was instructed by the court to gather information on "the degree of humiliation, dependence, and loss of dignity probably resulting from the condition and treatment."[32] This language reflects recognition that patients care about and may suffer from such elements as embarrassment and frustration from diminished intellectual functioning, frustration and helplessness from being dependent on others for every aspect of bodily functioning, humiliation from being viewed in a grossly debilitated state, rage at being physically restrained from removing life-sustaining equipment, or emotional pain in sensing a burden upon surrounding loved ones. Some patients, while competent, may even express their predilections about these considerations of impaired functioning and emotional suffering. Presumably, the majority opinion's mention of information about level of physical and cognitive functioning, as well as "humiliation, dependence, and loss of dignity," was intended to encourage implementation of the patient's predilections in this direction, at least where the expressions are clear enough to meet the subjective test.

Under the limited objective test, the first approach to best interests, the majority noted that the "same types of medical evidence" as in the case of the subjective test should be gathered. The court made specific reference to consideration of "level of functioning, degree of humiliation and dependency."[33] This could be interpreted as allowing a surrogate decision-maker to consider elements of helplessness, dependency, or embarrassment of the incompetent patient—at least where the prior expressions or patterns of conduct of the patient indicate that these elements are important to the patient. (The "limited-objective" test, it will be remembered, is triggered by "some trustworthy evidence" that the patient would have refused life-preserving treatment under the circumstances now confronted.)

This analysis would help explain the difference between assessing net benefits and burdens under the "limited-objective" as opposed to the "pure objective" test. Under the latter standard, the decision-maker (operating without any significant indication of patient wishes) might be confined to considerations of physical pain. Under the former, the decision-maker would consider emotional suffering or a minimum acceptable level of functioning as indicated by the patient's prior expressions and conduct.

On the other hand, "pain" in *Conroy* might have been intended to relate exclusively to physical pain. It would be easy to understand why the court was confining its consideration of best interests to physical pain and suffering. The court was intent on protecting "socially isolated and defenseless people suffering from physical or mental handicaps."[34] The court wished to be conservative in light of the monumental consequence involved—death of a helpless patient. The majority noted that limited function or a marginal "quality" of existence does not necessarily mean that it is in a person's best interests to die, even when the existence is projected to terminate in less than a year. The court was also well aware of the difficulties in accurately assessing both the physical and emotional benefits and burdens entailed in the life of an incompetent, noncommunicative patient. The court may therefore have wished to confine terminal decisions on behalf of nursing home patients—at least those who have not given any clearcut indication of their predilections—to situations where the incompetent patient is suffering intolerable physical pain.

It would be far preferable to interpret "pain and suffering" under the limited objective strand of the best interests test as including both physical and emotional pain, while confining the "severe pain" of the pure objective test to physical pain. This dichotomy would help underline the distinction between patients who were competent adults before their loss of faculties, as opposed to patients who have never been competent. This latter category includes persons who from birth or childhood have been severely retarded or insane. Once-competent patients, unlike never competent patients, may have provided expressions and patterns of conduct from which their personal predilections about emotional suffering or tolerable levels of functioning might be gleaned. For the patient who has always been severely retarded and noncommunicative, notions of emotional suffering may simply be out of place, or at least undeterminable with sufficient certainty. This latter class of patients will be discussed in chapter 4.

All in all, it would be desirable to permit consideration of emotional suffering in all cases—whether or not the patient had previously signalled (through prior expressions and conduct) the subjective importance of such elements as helplessness, dependence, and diminished capacity. Such elements of emotional suffering may be present even if the patient has not left "trustworthy evidence" of subjective wishes. The problem lies in detecting and measuring the presence and extent of such feelings as frustration, embarrassment, and humiliation in patients whose deteriorated condition prevents communication of their actual feelings.

Allowing consideration of emotional suffering and acceptable (to the patient) levels of functioning in assessing the best interests of once-competent patients still makes sense in many instances. If unremitting physical pain were a prerequisite to termination of life-preserving treatment (in the absence of clearcut prior instructions), even the permanently comatose and insensate individual would have to be maintained—a result inconsistent with the *Quinlan* decision itself. Moreover, the reality is that some deteriorating patients undergo extreme emotional suffering during the dying process. Feelings of helplessness, dependency, embarrassment, humiliation, and sense of burden may plague certain individuals,[35] and may be detectable even if the patient lacks sufficient capacity to be considered a competent patient. That is, patients reach various levels of incompetence, and at some levels it is still possible to perceive real, negative feelings plaguing the patient. Several recent sources therefore accept emotional suffering, and related notions of level of functioning and quality of existence,[36] as relevant factors in measuring the best interests of an incompetent patient whose own predilections (based on prior expressions) cannot reliably be discerned.[37]

It is worth repeating that the quality of salvageable existence is often an important factor in the proper handling of the dying, incompetent patient. Mitigation of suffering is a prime objective. That in turn involves, I have argued, consideration of the constancy and degree of both physical pain and emotional suffering. Relevant elements of emotional suffering (such as dependency, helplessness, or humiliation) are determined in part by the patient's "quality of life"—in terms of an expected level of physical and mental functioning. That is, feelings of dependence or helplessness are affected by the patient's capacity to function in his or her accustomed ways. Feelings of embarrassment are shaped in part by the patient's degree of pride in appearance and front presented to the world.

Mention of quality of life considerations in the death and dying context prompts some commentators to assert that the door will be opened to basing terminal decisions on "social worth" of individuals. The implication is that once the concept of a life "not worth living" is accepted, a variety of populations, including the retarded, insane, senile, or handicapped will be subject to abuse. The opinion in *Conroy* takes pains, therefore, to dispel any notion that decision-making may be based on social utility or personal worth assessments. Quality of life is deemed relevant only from the perspective of the patient, assessing benefits and burdens *to the patient* in order to avoid prolonging the dying process when no net benefit to the patient is forthcoming. Material societal concerns—the potential lack of productivity or economic burden stemming from maintenance of a gravely deteriorated person—are not compatible with *Conroy*'s definition of best interests of the patient.

This focus on the best interests of the patient ostensibly operates to also exclude such items as emotional and financial burdens to the surrounding family—at least where the patient has not clearly articulated a desire to have such elements included in the decision-making calculus. Yet it is extremely hard to divorce the family's suffering from the setting of a dying patient. This subject of emotional and economic burdens upon loved ones posed by protracted terminal care is a controversial one and will be dealt with separately.

Even with the allowance of emotional suffering as a relevant factor, only in extreme cases can it be said, with confidence, that withdrawal of life support is in the best interests of an incompetent person. As the *Conroy* opinion demonstrates, the vast majority of senile, severely impaired elderly patients cannot be said to be better off dead than alive. This is particularly so when viewed from the perspective of the feelings of the incompetent patient. Many such patients reach a stage at which they are essentially noncommunicative and largely insensate. For those patients, and other seriously incompetent persons, assessing their temporal feelings—either physical or emotional and either painful or positive—may be an impossible task.

Claire Conroy provides an illustration. While not brain dead or comatose, she was severely demented and could not communicate. Although two physicians testified as to her mental status, the evidence about her capacity to experience pain—let alone the intensity and duration of such pain—was deemed "inconclusive."[38] Though Ms. Conroy would occasionally moan when moved or fed, and would occasionally pull at her bandages and tubes, the court drew no conclusions from this conduct. Possible discomfort associated with the naso-gastric tube, or negative reaction to the restraints sometimes used to prevent her from interfering with the tube, had not been explored in the trial court. In short, her level of temporal suffering was by no means clear.

Ms. Conroy's capacity to experience pleasure or satisfaction was equally unclear. Her eyes sometimes followed persons in the room, and she "smiled on occasion when her hair was combed, or when she received a comforting rub." But she was unable to respond to verbal stimuli and one physician opined that she "had no higher functioning or consciousness."[39] In sum, it was difficult to say from the record in *Conroy* to what extent Ms. Conroy was really experiencing physical or emotional distress (or pleasure) in her lingering, debilitated state. The New Jersey Supreme Court therefore refused to say, based on the record, whether the attempt to remove Ms. Conroy's nourishment was in her best interests.

A major problem, then, in administering a best interests standard geared to the temporal physical and mental pain of an incompetent patient is that such suffering (or countervailing positive feelings) may be largely undeterminable. Under the current status of neurology and medical technology, it may be simply impossible to assess the temporal feelings—positive or negative—of a lingering, semi-comatose patient like Ms. Conroy.[40] Measurement of pain is extremely problematical, as pain is a complex phenomenon involving physiological, psychological, and cultural components. It is a personal, private sensation as to which there are no reliable physiological devices or measures. "Only [the patient] knows when it hurts, how much it hurts, or when the pain is relieved."[41] The patient may well be too incompetent to communicate actual feelings.

Nor is the patient's conduct a reliable index of physical or emotional feelings when the patient is operating at a low level of mentation. When patients pull at their life-sustaining tubes, as did Ms. Conroy, there is a temptation to regard the action as an expression of suffering and of a wish to be let alone, or even a plea to be allowed to die. Indeed, that *might* be the intended message. However the action might merely represent annoyance flowing in part from incomprehension of the purpose of the bodily invasion. Even a smile, as when Ms. Conroy received a hair comb or rub, is enigmatic in the context of very uncomprehending patients. It could be an expression of physical pleasure, or it could be an effort to communicate gratitude for an effort to comfort the patient, even though the effort had been unavailing from the patient's perspective.

The *Conroy* court's response to uncertainty about the distress being experienced by the virtually insensate, moribund patient was to demand more information. Had Ms. Conroy still been alive, the court would have remanded for additional medical evidence as to her pain and suffering, and more testimony about her personal beliefs and attitudes.[42] (This request for further information was consistent with the court's effort to apply a best interests approach accomodating both relief from unremitting suffering and attention to patient preferences.) In the absence of such additional proofs, the New Jersey Supreme Court would not endorse removal of the feeding tube as being in Ms. Conroy's best interests. The automatic course would then be preservation of the patient's lingering existence.

Perhaps the New Jersey Supreme Court's conclusion about Ms. Conroy's best interests was correct. Perhaps that conclusion was dictated by solicitude for the well being of debilitated, isolated, and institutionalized individuals. Yet a few other courts have shown a willingness to allow termination of life-preserving treatment for incompetent patients in a deteriorated state such as Ms. Conroy's.[43] An important question is whether the New Jersey Supreme Court's conclusion about Ms. Conroy's fate is consistent with its avowed effort to assure "humane" treatment for the institutionalized, severely impaired, dying individual.

Death with Dignity—Beyond the Temporal Interests
of the Insensate Patient

As illustrated by the condition of Claire Conroy, it is difficult if not impossible to shape the medical approach to uncomprehending and uncommunicative patients upon their contemporaneous feelings of physical pain or emotional anguish. Those feelings are too often undeterminable. What may be determinable is the treatment a broad concensus of thinking and feeling persons would want for themselves if they were reduced to the status of Ms. Conroy. In other words, it may be possible to gradually discern acceptable societal norms of humane handling of moribund patients. Just as constitutional norms of personal privacy must be shaped by "the traditions and collective conscience of the people,"[44] so the common law of handling dying patients will be shaped by shared notions of how "we" citizens want to be treated at that critical juncture. That is, shared notions of human dignity will ultimately govern decision-making on behalf of incompetent moribund patients.

The seeds of this approach were sown in the *Quinlan* decision.[45] Though Ms. Quinlan was biologically alive—with her brain stem controlling body temperature, breathing, heart rate, swallowing, blinking, and reaction to noxious stimuli—the court determined that as a person with no chance of returning to a cognitive existence, she need not be kept alive.[46] The court could not have been relying on the feelings of the patient, as she was insensate. The *Quinlan* court also disavowed any reliance on Ms. Quinlan's previous expressions. The court's determination was grounded instead on the conviction that preservation of biological existence under the circumstances offered "neither human nor humane benefit." That conviction, in turn, was grounded on the perception that the vast majority of people faced with irreversible coma would choose death.[47] Relief from the irreversible limbo of coma was deemed humane, even though the patient could no longer sense any relief.

Several sources besides *Quinlan* reflect recognition that the basic object must always be to provide humane treatment to the dying, with the definition of "humane" shaped by broad based societal notions of human dignity. Justice Handler's partial dissent in *Conroy* affords one example. Justice Handler criticized the majority for undue focus on physical pain to the detriment of "a whole cluster of other human values that have a proper place" in weighing the fate of a moribund patient.[48] Justice Handler specifically refers to human dignity and "basic human moral values" as the missing ingredients.[49] He seeks to define "best interests" of an incompetent patient as including "a collection of values that society will impute to incompetent persons who cannot express their own preferences."[50] Similarly, the President's Commission has implicitly recognized the role of shared perceptions of human dignity in making decisions for incompetent, terminally ill patients. The Commission notes that where the patient's wishes can't be discerned, the patient may be presumed to desire "what most reasonable people would want in similar circumstances."[51]

The challenge now is to lend content to the guiding principles of human dignity and humane treatment. Humane treatment is, by itself, an amorphous concept. Some people might regard life in a nursing home as itself undignified and degrading. As the New Jersey Supreme Court emphasized in *Conroy,* care must constantly be taken to safeguard defenseless beings against abuse.

As a starting point, perceptions about human dignity must be widely held before they can be implemented. Even widely shared perceptions must be examined critically. Seemingly enlightened societies have been known to accept slavery, witch hunts, and even genocide.

With all that in mind, I foresee that the basic guide for handling incompetent, terminally ill patients (at least those who have previously been competent) will eventually be "human dignity and humane treatment." Moreover, the key to that guideline will be how a strong majority of competent people would want themselves to be treated in the circumstances now confronting the moribund patient. This broad concensus will serve as an important index of "human dignity," subject always to the pervasive notion in Anglo-American jurisprudence that the state has a parens patriae obligation to protect helpless individuals against abuse and mistreatment. While broad concensus about human dignity in the dying process can serve as a strong indication of a morally acceptable approach, any concensus must still be subjected to judicial as well as legislative scrutiny of its moral base.

All this does not mean that private decision-makers or reviewing courts must commission public opinion polls to determine whether particular cases fall within common understanding of human dignity and humane treatment. The initial decision to terminate will be grounded on a guardian's perception of common human dignity, as tested and confirmed by a physician, the patient's family, and a public advocate (for those jurisdictions which adopt the procedures of *Conroy*). On some occasions, one source or another will object (sometimes a complaint emanates from hospital personnel, sometimes from a dissenting family member), and a judicial assessment will be rendered. The judicial assessment—as to whether a particular termination decision conforms to humane treatment—will examine evolving practices in institutions, as well as any other evidence of what human dignity requires or forbids. This judicial examination can include input by ethicists, philosophers, and clergy, among others. Gradually, classes of cases will crystallize and be reported, as has already occurred with regard to the permanently comatose patient.[52] People who are fearful of being handled pursuant to such a loose standard as human dignity and humane treatment, or people who wish to cling to the last possible moment of existence regardless of any indignities, can specify their wishes in advance and those wishes will be respected.

No one can precisely define the bounds of humane treatment, but I think I can describe some of the established principles of human dignity applicable in the death and dying context. I can also suggest some of the critical questions, even if I can't supply more than tentative answers.

Fulfillment of the Patient's Wishes

Respect for self-determination as an element of human dignity demands fulfillment of the patient's (competently expressed) preferences regarding medical intervention in the dying process. This is true whether the patient's prerogative is grounded in constitutional privacy or common law notions of bodily integrity and self-determination. It is so whether the decision-making formula is branded "substituted judgment," "limited objective," or just plain "best interests."

Of course, self-determination is based on notions of volition and choice. This normally means a considered judgment about the options and consequences of a decision. When the incompetent patient's wishes about death and dying have not been clearly expressed, it is appropriate to examine the patient's prior values, beliefs, and conduct for guidance. That examination of beliefs and patterns of conduct can offer insights into what the incompetent patient may be feeling in terms of emotional upset, or into the level of disfunction which the patient would regard as inconsistent with his own perception of human dignity. The more oblique or distant the patient's expressions or behavior, the more decision-makers must consider what course of treatment common human dignity suggests under the circumstances. At least some notions of human dignity have already crystallized and won widespread recognition within American society.

Relief from a Painful Dying Process

In striving to establish guidelines for "humane actions" toward incompetent dying patients, relief from a painful dying process is a preeminent object. This reflects a common understanding that the vast majority of people would seek relief from irremediable, severe pain, at least where the prognosis about level of functioning is dim. There appears to be little disagreement that providing relief from severe pain is part of a humane approach to handling incompetent, dying patients.

Emotional pain, to the extent that it is measurable, is an appropriate factor for consideration. Helplessness and embarrassment may be as antithetical to human dignity as physical pain. The *Conroy* court's hesitancy to articulate this factor reflects the court's determination to build legal doctrine slowly and deliberately in this highly sensitive field.

Cognition as a Prerequisite of Human Dignity

In *Quinlan,* the New Jersey Supreme Court held that a permanently comatose individual could be removed from life-preserving machinery.

Since that decision, the highest state courts in at least five other jurisdictions have so ruled.[53] In addition, respected medical sources recognize that all means of life support may ethically be discontinued for a patient in an irreversible coma.[54]

The implicit judgment being made is that the permanent absence of mentation reduces human status to a level at which termination of life support is consistent with respect for human dignity. There have been some counter suggestions that termination of a person in a vegetative state is justified in order to relieve emotional and economic burdens on surrounding loved ones. I respectfully suggest that the most appropriate basis for termination of support to a permanently comatose patient is the shared perception that total lack of cognition, with the concomitant inability to interact with the environment and to relate to persons, represents a dismal status for a previously competent individual. At that point, the removal of life support is deemed consistent with human dignity and humane handling. Hence, the growing judicial and medical concensus that individuals need not be maintained in a hopeless limbo of permanent coma.

One unresolved question is whether people who are "semicomatose" can be similarly handled. There is limited and inconclusive judicial precedent on the issue.[55] Where the semicomatose condition includes a permanent absence of all cognitive function—that is, the brain cannot synthesize or understand outside stimuli—the result will probably be to allow life-preserving equipment to be removed, as in the case of the totally comatose patient.[56] Where there is some form of cognition remaining however, there is no common understanding that "humane" handling dictates termination of life-preserving treatment solely on the ground of low level of mentation.

The trial court in *Conroy* emphasized the "virtually zero intellectual level" of Claire Conroy in authorizing the removal of nourishment.[57] Yet the New Jersey Supreme Court was unwilling to rely on her intellectual level as a basis for termination. Medical practice appears to be evolving in the direction of withholding medical intervention, including artificial feeding, from the "severely demented" patient only when the patient is facing death within a short period.[58]

It would appear that so long as a patient is intellectually capable of interacting with his or her environment at anything more than a pure reflex level, there is no concensus that low intellectual function, by itself, warrants removal of life-support as part of a humane approach to terminal care. Thus, an insane or retarded person may not be singled out on the basis of low intellectual function and given less vigorous care. A further question is the significance of reduced intellectual function, along with other elements of disfunction, in assessment of the previously competent patient's overall deteriorated status for purposes of deciding what treatment respect for human dignity dictates.

Degradation in the Dying Process

The central question regarding patients in the deteriorated status of Ms. Conroy is what human dignity requires for a formerly active, independent, and articulate person. Is there a broad community concensus that total immobility, along with virtually total incomprehension and noncommunication, represents a gross degradation for such a person in the face of an inexorably approaching death? Certainly, there are some persons who would consider the total disfunction, helplessness, and dependence to be a humiliating condition. An articulate being is reduced to a periodic moaning sound. An active individual is reduced to total immobility, curled permanently in a semi-fetal position. An independent person lies totally dependent on others for every bodily function from nourishment to removal of bodily wastes. A social being has permanently lost the capacity to relate to others. I, for one, have no trouble agreeing with Ms. Conroy's nephew that the time had come to offer a humane escape. If there is, as suggested above, broad concensus that permanent coma is a dehumanizing limbo, there should eventually be broad concensus that Ms. Conroy's nephew's proposed course of action was respectful of human dignity.[59]

Another dimension of degradation, not fully explored in *Conroy*,[60] is the use of physical restraints to prevent an incompetent patient from tampering with life-sustaining equipment. Presence of such restraints has potential significance in at least two ways. First, it is an indication of annoyance or distaste by the patient—a factor which is relevant to assessing the patient's degree of suffering.[61] Second, at least where a patient must be trussed up for protracted periods—as where the patient is resisting an implanted nourishment tube or attachment to a dialysis machine—the physical restraint might be regarded as an assault on human dignity. Even when the object is to keep a patient alive, there is a distasteful aspect in protracted physical restraint of a resisting patient.[62]

There may be some temptation to claim that notions of humiliation or dependence are not relevant to patients such as Ms. Conroy. Either the patient is totally unaware and uncomprehending, or the extent of emotional discomfort is undeterminable. Nonetheless, as previously noted, there are good reasons for sparing persons degradation even if they can't sense the degradation at the moment it occurs. It is useful for every citizen to know that in the event he or she is incompetent during the dying process, human dignity will be respected. If the vast majority of competent persons regard reduction to total helplessness, dependency, and disfunction as a degrading spectre which will soil their memory, then the proposed removal of Ms. Conroy's naso-gastric tube would appear to be humane.

A further objection might be that if such a spectre is in fact distasteful, any competent person can provide for such a contingency by leaving instructions. The reality is that most persons will not utilize that route because of unwillingness to seriously confront their mortality. It is also difficult to anticipate and detail in advance the combination of factors which any particular individual might regard as warranting termination of treatment. The variables are many, including physical impairment, mental disfunction, chances of remission, chances of a miraculous cure, physical pain, emotional suffering, expense, emotional toll on those surviving, etc. Even if an attempt is made to spell out in advance the level of functioning acceptable to the individual, there is no assurance that the instructions will be accessible at the critical moment—given the mobility of the population. If there is truly concensus that humane handling dictates that a patient like Ms. Conroy be allowed to expire, a conscientious guardian ought to be permitted to follow that course.

IV

TROUBLE SPOTS ON THE HORIZON

Supplanting the Guardian's Decision

Sometimes, primary decision-makers acting on behalf of an incompetent dying patient insist that "everything possible be done" to preserve the patient, no matter how dismal the patient's condition. The motive will likely be salutary. The decision-maker may simply be "hoping for a miracle" and therefore refuse to take any step, such as removal of a respirator or cessation of artificial nourishment, which will accelerate the lingering patient's death. Yet if the dying patient has reached a point of deterioration where no benefit to the patient is forthcoming and chances of recovery are nil (within the limits of medical certainty), continued maintenance may appear to be either "inhumane" or inconsistent with the "best interests" of the incompetent patient. At the same time, considerable resources in terms of time and equipment may be being devoted to the languishing patient. Is it conceivable that steps will be taken to supplant the guardian's determination to maintain the patient? Is it conceivable that funding sources will refuse to continue footing the bill for maintenance?

The permanently comatose patient may provide an illustration. It is now judicially established that such a patient *may* be removed from life-preserving equipment, sometimes according to a substituted judgment standard and sometimes pursuant to a best interests test. But *must* such a patient be removed? The *New York Times* recently described a sixty-one-year-old woman languishing in a vegetative state in a New York hospital and being maintained on kidney dialysis treatment at an annual cost of $22,000. Of her five children responsible for initial decision-making, the four "who never visited her" favored maintaining the treatment. The newspaper article reported that a psychiatrist was scheduled to meet with the family in an effort to have them reconsider their position. The psychiatrist observed: "If they're so concerned, they should see her in this awful vegetative state that we can prolong indefinitely at immense cost for what gain."[1] The *Times* also recently described a "six-million-dollar woman," a permanently comatose patient who had been maintained in that state for eighteen years, with accumulating costs from a long list of medical specialties including neurology, neurosurgery, urology, gynecology, dermatology, and radiology.[2] And, of course, a comatose Karen Ann Quinlan was maintained on artificial nourishment (though not antibiotics) for over nine years after her respirator was removed in the belief that she would quickly expire. The annual cost to taxpayers was approximately $32,000. At the moment that Ms. Quinlan died in June 1985, there were seventy-four comatose patients whose care was being subsidized by Medicaid in New Jersey.[3]

Standards of review of a guardian's terminal decision are beginning to be shaped by the courts. Where the responsible decision-maker makes a choice to terminate life-preserving care, that choice will likely be respected so long as it is made in good faith and within the bounds of reasonableness. That is, there is a clear trend to defer to conscientious decision-makers' appraisals of a dying patient's subjective preferences or best interests, so long as the particular decision has a plausible basis under the circumstances.[4] Two elements are required. The decision must be taken in subjective good faith—that is, without any intention to harm the moribund patient. Further, the determination must be grounded on some objective facts such that a reasonable person could find that the patient would have desired termination of treatment, or that termination would be in the patient's best interests, or that termination would be consistent with the humane handling of an incompetent patient, depending on the decision-making standard employed in the particular jurisdiction.

Presumably, a similar deferential standard prevails in reviewing a guardian's determination to *continue* life-preserving machinery for a waning patient. That is, so long as a reasonable person could conclude that continued maintenance is consistent with a dying patient's wishes and/or best interests, the guardian's decision will not normally be overridden by a court or any other agency. Under that approach, even a decision to maintain a permanently comatose patient would not be subject to being supplanted. Given the inherent uncertainty of medical prognosis, preserving a faint chance for a medical miracle cannot be viewed as totally unreasonable. Since the comatose patient is not suffering in the limbo being maintained, it cannot be said at this stage in the evolution of relevant mores that preservation is "inhumane." If the moribund patient is enduring unrelievable suffering, the chances of overriding the guardian's determination are greater. There is still no judicial precedent on this, though, and courts will be hesitant to supplant a guardian's conscientious belief that some life, even though ostensibly torturous, is preferable to nonexistence.

The one instance in which a guardian's decision to preserve an incompetent patient *ought* to be overridable—though again there is as yet no precedent available—is where the patient's previously expressed wishes are clearly being contravened. Those wishes reflect a decision to resist life-preserving medical intervention—an exercise of autonomy with a strong common law and constitutional grounding. Of course, there will be disputes about the proximity and clarity of the patient's instructions, and about the possibility of changed circumstances which the patient will be alleged not to have anticipated. Nonetheless, if a court finds that the decision-maker is violating the patient's prior determination, the decision-maker should be relieved of responsibility. This is so even in the case of aberrational wishes, for the patient's autonomy includes the prerogative to make "unwise" decisions.

Of course, once a patient's condition meets the legal definition of death, it is no longer appropriate to continue pumping air or nutrients into the corpse. Evolving definitions of death however won't solve the issue of most long-term patients being maintained in comatose or semi-comatose states. Though the overwhelming majority of American jurisdictions have moved or are moving to a "brain-death" test of death, most victims of irreversible coma don't satisfy that definition. Persons in irreversible coma have generally lost operation of their "upper" brain, which controls thinking and awareness, but their brain stem or lower brain continues to function and control certain mechanical functions of the body. Their EEG (measurement of brain activity) does not register totally flat. The brain-death definition, by contrast, requires total brain death, not just destruction of the upper brain.[5] In short, a person in irreversible coma whose brain stem continues to function is not legally dead.

A number of sources have argued that a permanently comatose patient—lacking awareness, thinking capacity, and the ability to relate to other beings—lacks minimum status for personhood and ought to be considered as dead. The thesis is that life can have no further meaning for the patient without at least partial consciousness. Human status assertedly requires some capacity to experience an environment and to relate to others. Without appreciation of human experience, the patient's status is regarded as mere biological existence.

Yet no societal concensus exists that deterioration to mere biological existence renders a former human being nonhuman. Moreover, there is considerable concern about the implications of such a position for severely retarded or brain-damaged beings. There is no reliable physiological measure of what constitutes human personality or personhood. Without such a reliable index, there is reluctance to start redefining personhood even though *total* absence of consciousness does indeed reflect an absence of customary human attributes such as awareness and capacity to relate to others. Some commentators argue that once a single brick is removed from the dam protecting the sanctity of all life, the entire dam is liable to collapse and every life is at risk.[6] While this may be hyperbole, the principle is sound that redefinition of personhood according to intellectual capacity can proceed only when clear lines and societal concensus are obtained.

In sum, a guardian's decision to continue maintenance of a waning patient—even a permanently comatose one—does not normally constitute either abuse of discretion or abuse of a corpse. So long as the patient is not grievously suffering, and so long as the guardian is not contravening any prior instructions from the previously competent patient, the decision to preserve existence is probably consistent with guardianship principles. Nonetheless, when no material benefit is derived by the patient, as where a patient is being maintained in a permanent vegetative state, there is serious question whether public funding sources should continue to absorb the considerable economic costs involved.

Government health benefit programs have always shown some sensitivity to allocation of societal resources. Medicaid, for example, would not finance an expensive procedure yielding marginal returns—such as an artificial heart implantation. Indeed, it took special legislation to impel the public funding of kidney dialysis treatment despite the obvious benefits deriving from that form of therapy. It is only a matter of time, then, before public funding sources rebel at the considerable sums expended to sustain patients for whom no benefits are apparent other than biological existence. One gerontology expert observed in January 1985: "Cost has to be a factor. We have to avoid misallocation of high technology to individuals who have no likelihood of benefitting from them."[7]

The argument is not simply that the money could be better spent elsewhere. A claim could always be made that resources would be better spent in preventive medicine than in acute care or chronic care for severely retarded or terribly senile individuals. Or that aerospace research would be a wiser use of societal resources than preserving marginal existences. Ordinarily, for purposes of health care funding we don't try to weigh lives, at least not lives of defined groups or categories of patients, against potential societal benefits if the health funding were diverted elsewhere. Not only is there a problem of comparing apples with oranges, but there is no assurance that liberated funds would be allocated in any particularly constructive way.[8]

The argument is that public funds ought not to be expended for patients deriving no material benefit from the procedures being funded. The recent President's Commission, for example, recognized that society is not obligated to support every medical intervention and that excessive cost in relation to limited benefits for the patient may shape the limits of public funding responsibility.[9] That argument will eventually prevail, so long as reimbursement guidelines can be devised which don't jeopardize efforts to preserve patients still receiving benefit from treatment. The permanently comatose patient seems to offer a reasonably clear dividing line. Thus, while a guardian may continue to seek maintenance of a person in a permanent vegetative existence, public funding sources will eventually refuse to finance such care. Medical institutions will likely be unwilling to pick up the resulting economic burden where the patient's or family's resources are insufficient to keep funding the maintenance being provided.[10]

Some sources assert that the pressure to reduce expenditures for terminal care has already begun on the part of public funding sources. The contention is that reimbursement schemes based on fixed rates according to a patient's diagnosis (called diagnosis related groups, or DRG's) already provide an incentive for health care providers to cut corners in care and to shorten protracted hospitalizations. In the case of dying patients, this reimbursement policy is alleged to impel diminished willingness to provide expensive life-sustaining services.[11]

Survivors' Interests, Economic Costs, and Patients' Altruism

Surrounding family and friends are sometimes subjected to severe emotional and economic strain during a loved one's prolonged dying process. Many persons want to spare their survivors such suffering. A competent patient can direct his own terminal care accordingly, and can presumably leave explicit directions on the subject to help guide a proxy decision-maker after the patient becomes incompetent. Consideration of survivors' interests is also arguably appropriate where an incompetent patient previously exhibited particular warmth and affection for family and friends. This is true whether the standard being used to guide a decision-maker is "substituted judgment" or "best interests." If altruism is an established part of the character of the moribund patient, then solicitude for survivors may be appropriate in implementing that patient's self-defined best interests. Similarly, the substituted judgment doctrine would allow for consideration of survivors' interests where consistent with the patient's established character. Indeed, that legal doctrine was often used (in administering an incompetent person's property) to allow a guardian to bestow a gift upon a party to whom the incompetent had no legal obligation.[12]

The harder question is whether a guardian can assume a modicum of altruism on the part of a patient even in the absence of previously demonstrated concern for survivors' interests. The President's Commission was apparently willing to attribute to incompetent patients a desire to mitigate burdens on those surrounding them. Their recent report commented:

> The impact of a decision on an incapacitated patient's loved ones may be taken into account in determining someone's best interests, for most people do have an important interest in the well-being of their families or close associates.[13]

Some courts have indicated that concern for survivors' interests is part of the reason why removal of a permanently comatose patient's life-preserving equipment is deemed to be in that patient's interests.[14]

Not everyone is willing to say that such altruism is an innate human characteristic. It is also conceivable that altruism is grounded in the sense of satisfaction which the altruist receives, an experience that may elude the incompetent patient at the moment that a surrogate decision-maker acts to terminate care. While I have argued that it is fair to impute to an incompetent patient a wish to be treated "humanely," I'm not yet convinced that the imputed humanity should automatically include a willingness to have survivors' economic and emotional strains considered in shaping the medical treatment of a dying patient. Moreover, insertion of survivors' interests into the decision-making framework begins to smack of the kinds of social utility considerations which are anathema in the context of handling dying patients.[15] Suddenly patients' lives are being weighed (at least in part) against discomforts and strains being undergone by others. It is hard enough to balance the benefits and burdens to the patient without bringing in outside interests such as emotional strains on the family. Moreover, there is a potential conflict of interest created when survivors' interests are made a regular factor in the decision-making calculus. As we will see in the next chapter, those very survivors, the immediate family, will likely have an important role in the decision-making process. For all the above reasons, a consideration of the survivors' emotional well-being should probably only enter into a guardian's calculus in response to the patient's previously articulated wishes, or clearly established character trait.

On the other hand, it is naive to think that decision-makers will be oblivious to the resources—physical, emotional, and monetary—being devoted to a dying patient who has reached extreme debilitation and has no prospect of regaining a healthful existence. Physicians, for example, are well aware of the constraints that are placed on their attention to other patients, as well as the strains on the surviving family by terminal care. Thus, a recent report published by a group of respected medical experts in the prestigious New England Journal of Medicine recommended with respect to handling of the hopelessly ill patients: "Financial ruin of the patient's family, as well as the drain on resources for treatment of other patients who are not hopelessly ill, should be weighed . . ., although the patient's welfare obviously remains paramount."[16] Consistent with this position, the AMA Judicial Council has ruled that in making treatment decisions for severely deteriorated adult patients, "the *primary* consideration should be what is best for the individual patient and not the avoidance of a burden to the family or to society."[17] Under these approaches, the principle guideline is always preservation of life, so long as that is possible under "humane" conditions; but room is left for consideration of the burdens on others where the patient's condition is marginal.[18]

The economic burden of terminal care is evident. Most people die in expensive acute care hospitals geared to sophisticated medical intervention rather than the supportive handling (nursing-type services) appropriate to the needs of many dying patients. An informal study in June 1984 of 143 deaths in a New York City hospital disclosed that the average cost of the final hospitalization was $15,000.[19] That is an average figure. Some terminal bouts are much more expensive. Insurance and/or public funding may cover much, but by no means all of the expenses. In short, the cost element looms over the decision-making process even if it is not enumerated as a factor.

In theory, economic burdens ought to remain divorced from terminal decision-making. Society (taxpayers' funds) should assume all fiscal burdens associated with maintaining poor or uninsured incompetent patients whose lives are being preserved, and who arguably derive some benefit from that preservation.[20] But the reality is that survivors and treating institutions are sometimes left holding the bag, or empty purse. Consequently, survivors' burdens will remain a lurking omnipresence, at least a subconscious factor in the effort to shape appropriate treatment for the incompetent, dying individual.

Some sources recognize economic realities and suggest that the financial cost of terminal care can properly be a conscious factor in decision-making. For example, Roman Catholic doctrine currently allows a "proportionality" principle to govern choice of medical treatment for the terminally ill. Cost of treatment may be considered in relation to limited benefits obtainable because of the patient's poor condition and prognosis. It is permissible under that approach to act out of "a desire not to impose excessive expense on the family or the community."[21]

Nonetheless, there does not yet seem to be a broad concensus that survivors' economic interests should be a routine part of the standard for deciding an incompetent patient's fate. Survivors' economic (as well as emotional) burdens may explicitly be considered in response to the patient's manifest preferences indicated while the patient was competent. But where the patient's preferences are not discernible, and the patient's own best interests and/or humane handling become the guides, survivors' strains cannot properly come into play, at least not under any standard of guardian's responsibility that has as yet been judicially endorsed.

I have previously suggested that public funding sources will impose restraints on the provision of care for dying medical patients.[22] These restraints will probably take the form of refusals by public funding sources to subsidize particularly expensive processes (such as heart transplants), or to pay for maintenance of classes of patients who derive no benefit from care (such as the permanently comatose). When this occurs, there will be an indirect but clear impact on treatment options concerning incompetent patients. In the absence of public funding, the institution providing care may be unwilling to absorb the continuing costs. The costs of life-preserving care then willy-nilly enter the picture.

Next of kin and other surrounding relatives will inevitably be made aware of financial pressures flowing from the absence of public funding. The next of kin will probably be asked by the care-providing institution to pick up the economic burden. But only a spouse is legally obligated to bear the costs of "necessities" provided to an incompetent, adult patient. Even if a spouse is deemed legally responsible for the well-being of an incompetent patient, the economic burden which a spouse would be expected to undertake is limited. A spouse is not required to pauperize himself or herself in order to provide even life-preserving medical care. Not many spouses, for example, would be in an economic situation in which they would be expected to fund an artificial heart in order to extend the survival of a moribund patient. But even if the spouse's financial responsibility is limited (from a legal perspective), that spouse can hardly avoid feeling in a moral bind if the care-providing institution approaches and requests assurance that the life-preserving costs will be reimbursed.

More distant relatives don't have any legal responsibility toward financially maintaining an adult, incompetent patient. Yet when public fund-ing ceases, and the care-providing institution expresses unwillingness to absorb the resulting economic burden, the nonspouse relative is inevita-bly aware of financial considerations at the moment of making medical decisions on behalf of an incompetent patient. While the care-providing institution will probably not threaten to evict the moribund patient, there will likely be pressures on the relatives to agree to pick up the costs or to make arrangements with another institution to continue the care. Under the AMA Judicial Council position described above, the cost element may consciously be considered, at least when the patient's wel-fare (always the governing factor) doesn't demand preservation of medi-cal care. If the patient's best interests dictate maintenance of treatment, the decision-makers' obligation would appear to be to resist any institu-tional efforts to cease treatment and to remind the institution of their undertaking not to harm a helpless patient in dire need of continued medical assistance. How such a plea will fare in the case of patients needing particularly expensive care remains to be seen.

The Never-Competent Patient

Some persons have lacked the mental capacity to make significant decisions for themselves from birth or early childhood. They are vari-ously referred to as the congenitally incompetent or never-competent. I'll use the latter term. For such persons, every medical decision has and always will require a surrogate decision-maker. The question here is how such a surrogate decision-maker must address life and death determina-tions involving the never-competent patient. The issue arises whenever the never-competent patient faces a potentially fatal condition—whether it be pneumonia, cancer, or cardiac arrest.[23]

As all the decision-making standards previously discussed are aimed at affording incompetent patients human dignity, and as never-competent patients are human beings, there is a temptation to simply transfer the regular standards to this setting. Yet any standard grounded on auton-omy and self-determination may not be applicable in the context of never-competent patients. And, because we are dealing with largely noncomprehending and noncommunicative individuals, their "best in-terests" may also be particularly difficult to gauge. Finally, human dignity may not mean precisely the same thing for a never-competent patient as for a previously competent patient.

The *Saikewicz* case[24] in Massachusetts provides a vivid illustration of the complexities involved. That 1977 decision by the highest state court in Massachusetts was important because it was the first major decision extending the *Quinlan* principle—that life-preserving medical treatment can sometimes be withheld or withdrawn from an incompetent patient— to a noncomatose, fully conscious individual. It was also important because it dealt with a never-competent person.

Joseph Saikewicz was a sixty-seven-year-old resident of a state institution for handicapped persons. He had resided in that institution for over fifty years. Saikewicz was and had always been profoundly mentally retarded. He had an I.Q. of ten and a mental age of approximately two years and eight months. He was totally nonverbal and could communicate only through gestures and grunts. He could not respond intelligibly to inquiries whether he was experiencing pain. He had been mobile and physically healthy up until April 1976 when he was stricken with a form of leukemia that is inevitably fatal. The issue then became whether to administer chemotherapy to Mr. Saikewicz.

If chemotherapy were given to Saikewicz (via an intravenous tube over the course of several weeks), there would be a thirty to forty percent chance of a remission which would last from two to thirteen months. The treatment would entail certain side effects—nausea, numbness, bladder irritation, and probably bleeding or infection requiring blood transfusions. In addition, Mr. Saikewicz would probably resist the intravenous line and would have to be physically restrained during I.V. administrations. If left untreated, Mr. Saikewicz would die within a few months without experiencing significant discomfort or pain.

The superintendent of the Massachusetts institution housing Mr. Saikewicz sought judicial guidance as to whether chemotherapy should be given. The lower court judge ruled in May 1976 that "the negative factors of treatment exceeded the benefits" and therefore ordered that no treatment be administered other than "supportive measures" to make the patient comfortable.[25] In July 1976, the Supreme Judicial Court of Massachusetts upheld this order and Mr. Saikewicz died in September 1976 without pain or discomfort. In its ruling, the Massachusetts high court sought to shape the standards which ought to govern treatment decisions for incompetent patients such as Mr. Saikewicz. Like *Quinlan*, which preceded it by only a few months, *Saikewicz* has had a wide impact and deserves careful examination.

The Supreme Judicial Court started from the premise that human dignity must be extended to an incompetent patient as it would be to a competent patient. A competent leukemia patient would be entitled to resist chemotherapy by exercising rights of privacy, bodily integrity, and self-determination. In order to respect the dignity and worth of the incompetent patient, the patient should therefore be afforded "the same panoply of rights and choices" as recognized in competent persons.[26] To accomplish that aim, the court ruled, a surrogate decision-maker should utilize a "substituted judgment" approach aimed at implementing the incompetent patient's actual interests and preferences. The basic object became to make the same decision Joseph Saikewicz would have made under the circumstances confronted.

As previously described, the substituted judgment standard seeks to implement the autonomy interest of an incompetent patient. In the context of a previously competent patient, the approach makes sense. The patient may have given instructions regarding his care, or at least have developed a mature person's value system or personality profile from which the patient's preferences could be gleaned. But Joseph Saikewicz was, in effect, a small child all his sixty-seven years, never capable of making judgments or expressing wishes which would be respected in medical decisions on his behalf. In the case of such a never-competent person, notions of free choice and autonomy simply have no place. Thus, the Supreme Judicial Court was misguided in attempting to apply a pure substituted judgment standard to the never-competent patient.

With the never-competent patient, the basic object remains to respect intrinsic human dignity. This is so even though the person has never possessed the mental capacity necessary for self-determination. The object is normally accomplished (for example, in the context of children) by seeking to make medical decisions in the "best interests" of the incompetent patient. In that way, benefits that might be chosen by a competent patient exercising self-determination can be accorded to a never-competent patient. This might occur, for example, regarding decisions on abortion or sterilization. By allowing such medical procedures on never-competent patients when in their best interests, courts promote the human dignity of such patients by affording access to beneficial results which competent patients could, and likely would, choose under similar circumstances.

As the Massachusetts courts fully recognized, a competent person could choose nontreatment in the face of a painful or torturous dying process. Such a nontreatment option should accordingly be available in the case of a never-competent patient where withholding of care would be in that patient's best interests. The main elements of the best interests test have already been outlined in the discussion of *Conroy,* above. Application of such a standard to guide decision-makers entails careful assessment of the various benefits and burdens available to the patient with treatment, versus without treatment. As discovered in *Conroy,* the best interests standard is difficult to apply to a formerly competent individual who has become totally noncommunicative and has never issued instructions about terminal treatment. It is even more difficult to apply in the context of a noncommunicative patient who has never been able to communicate feelings and preferences.

The best interests formula is sometimes identical with an effort to decide what a reasonable competent person in the incompetent's situation would want. For people are customarily assumed to choose what is in their best interests. Deciding what a reasonable, competent person would want is aided by an understanding of the patient's prior lifestyle and chosen patterns of behavior. But in the case of a never-competent patient, chosen lifestyle and autonomous behavior patterns are lacking.

The effort of the Massachusetts courts to assess the benefits and burdens involved in treatment of Joseph Saikewicz is illustrative of the difficulty of assessing a never-competent patient's best interests. Those courts purported to be acting, in choosing a course of nontreatment for Saikewicz, in light of his particularized interests. The basic determination was that the pain and suffering surrounding the side effects of chemotherapy would outweigh the benefit of possible extension of the patient's life for a period of between two and thirteen months. Yet, the courts conceded that most competent persons facing leukemia would choose to undergo the chemotherapy in spite of distasteful side effects. What supposedly distinguished Joseph Saikewicz was his inability to understand why he would be undergoing the treatment and accompanying side effects. That incomprehension would allegedly result in fear, confusion, and disorientation which would exacerbate the patient's discomfort or suffering.

The courts' calculus *might* be correct. It seems reasonable to think that an uncomprehending individual would feel enhanced discomfort because of incomprehension of the reasons for various medical interventions and noxious consequences. Yet normal assumptions about human patterns of feeling and emotion may not be fully applicable to a patient who has never had anything like normal mental functioning or normal socialization. Moreover, would the patient's suffering be increased (by noncomprehension) enough to justify foregoing a chance for a significant prolongation of existence? If Saikewicz could have been cured, wouldn't chemotherapy have been administered despite all his discomforts? What was being foregone by nontreatment was a thirty to forty percent chance for a remission—a period of 'normal' functioning—for between two and thirteen months. Perhaps the courts were tacitly saying that a chance for a two to thirteen month extension of his handicapped existence was not worth very much suffering. In any event, the case underlines the problems of assessing the feelings, pleasures, pains, and preferences of a patient who has an I.Q. of ten and has always operated at a reduced intellectual level.

The general situation in dealing with never-competent patients is even more complicated because decision-makers must cope with various degrees of both prior and present incompetence. There are wide ranges of mental impairment and not every incompetent patient operates at the dismal level of Joseph Saikewicz. Patients who are mentally incompetent to make informed decisions may still have strong adverse feelings about treatment which must be considered. There are a number of reported cases, for example, in which incompetent patients physically resisted medical interventions such as blood transfusions, intravenous medication, or surgical implantation of a feeding tube. The patients' actions can't be viewed as though they represented a competent, considered rejection of treatment. The patients may have been reacting instinctively to annoyances, or to confusion stemming from noncomprehension of the reasons for the interventions. At the same time, the patient's distaste for the intervention is relevant in assessing the benefits and burdens felt by the patient if treatment is continued.

I argued above that where temporal best interests of the incompetent patient are difficult to discern, considerations of human dignity and humane handling will eventually govern. But this notion of humane treatment is particularly problematical in the case of a never-competent patient. Simply put, dictates of human dignity may differ for a patient who has always been profoundly retarded as opposed to a patient who was once healthy and vigorous. Take the example of a patient who must be physically restrained in order to avoid tampering with feeding or medication tubes. To be sure, the never competent patient may feel frustration and resentment from having movement restricted, as would a previously competent patient. Further, there may be an intrinsic indignity in being trussed up or drugged for lengthy periods that is also applicable to the extremely debilitated, never-competent patient. Nonetheless, some elements of indignity may be totally absent in the case of the never-competent patient—for example, embarrassment from reduced capacity to function or humiliation from being totally dependent on other persons. In short, normal assumptions about human dignity may not be fully transferable to the never-competent patient.

This is not to say that basic human dignity is inapplicable to the never-competent patient. A certain core definition of human dignity will be applicable to all patients—whether previously competent or not. I am merely saying that the concept of human dignity might be somewhat different for some never-competent patients because certain elements of human dignity—such as a sense of embarrassment or humiliation—

might not be as acutely felt by certain never-competent persons. Ironically, the practical consequence of this conclusion might be that a dying,
never-competent patient would in certain instances be preserved longer
than a previously competent patient in identical circumstances. This is
because a decision-maker might not be able to say that the stage of
deterioration at which preservation of a previously competent patient
would be "inhumane" is the same for a never-competent patient. This
consequence flows in part from the natural effort of decision-makers to
shape the dying process according to the particularized situation of the
individual patient. Again, any consideration that qualifies as basic human
dignity must be applied to all patients regardless of whether they have
ever been competent.

Implications for the Institutionalized, Debilitated Population

This book has addressed various criteria for decision-making on behalf of incompetent patients—from substituted judgment to best
interests and beyond. Most of the situations contemplated have been
ones in which a patient has been stricken with an irreversible terminal
illness. In such situations, it is clear that medical intervention may sometimes be withheld or withdrawn in order to ease the dying process or to
carry out the wishes of a previously competent patient. Difficulties are
invariably faced in applying decision-making criteria to the infinite variety of fact patterns occurring, but the basic principles are discernible.

Harder issues arise in the context of highly debilitated, but nonter-
minally ill persons languishing in institutions. These might be severely
retarded individuals, or senile persons suffering from chronic but not
immediately life-threatening conditions. Can treatment be withheld
when various life-threatening diseases, such as pneumonia, set in? May a
nonresuscitation order (DNR) be entered on a patient's chart so the
patient will not be revived in the event of cardiac arrest? Can nutrition be
regarded as an aspect of medical support in this context and omitted
either before or after the onset of a potentially fatal condition?

Nursing homes, in which one and a quarter million Americans averag-
ing eighty-two-years-old are housed, offer one setting in which these
issues are regularly confronted. Some portion of residents in such institutions are highly debilitated, suffer physically or emotionally, and
face only a prospect of further deterioration and death. Treatment issues
then arise regarding such items as pneumonia, fluid loss associated with
diarrhea, antibiotics for bladder or other infections, and artificial feeding. It is increasingly clear that some nontreatment decisions are being

made in such institutions on the basis that the "life of a slowly declining resident is sufficiently painful or tragic that death appears to offer awaited release from suffering."[27]

At precisely what stage of deterioration can nontreatment orders, nonresuscitation orders, or cessation of artificial nourishment be instituted? The theoretical standards for decision-making must remain the same in this setting as those discussed in the context of irreversible terminal diseases—progressing from substituted judgment to best interests, and perhaps including human dignity. The further question is how these apply in practice.

Quality of existence—from the perspective of the patient's interests rather than a utilitarian perspective—remains an important concept. The concept should include physical and emotional pain, as well as loss of function resulting in a status degrading to a formerly competent patient's dignity. But there is no broad concensus that a particular level of mental functioning is a minimum level to justify administration of medical measures.

Some persons contend that an existence without capacity to read, write, and care for oneself is devoid of qualities necessary to meaningful life. Others assert that any human life must be preserved even if the being is nonsensient and lacks capacity to fulfill human nature by thinking and interacting. But neither of these extreme opinions appears to be widely held. There does appear to be a broad concensus that a person languishing in a permanent coma may be allowed to expire by removal of all forms of medical intervention including antibiotics and artificial nourishment. Within the last two years, several courts have upheld removal of intravenous tubes providing nutrition and hydration to a permanently comatose patient.[28] A recent report by respected medical authorities deemed it "morally justifiable to withhold antibiotics and artificial nutrition and hydration" from patients in a permanent vegetative state.[29]

Efforts to go further and to define a minimal "meaningful existence" in terms of mental awareness and ability to relate to others have not been accepted. That is, as long as the individual has some level of cognition, some consciousness of surroundings, there is no concensus that a low level of function, by itself, warrants termination of life support. Joseph Saikewicz, the sixty-seven-year-old with a mental age of two years and eight months, clearly functioned at a very primitive level. But he was conscious and had some cognizance of the world around him, and care could not be withheld based on his low intellectual capacity. Similarly, Claire Conroy operated at a "virtually zero" intellectual level, but her care could not be withdrawn on that basis alone.

All this does not mean that full medical intervention is always required for incompetent patients in chronic debilitated states up until the last stages of irreversible terminal illness. My own view is that there are rare instances where removal or withholding of medical intervention may indeed be justified for patients in extremely debilitated, though not immediately life-threatening states. First, there may be instances when patients' preincompetence expressions or patterns of behavior indicate that they would have resisted further assistance at the stage of debilitation now reached. Those expressions should be honored. Second, there may be instances when existence is marginal, and where emotional or physical suffering by the patient is discernible, to the extent that further measures to preserve existence, including antibiotics, can legitimately be omitted. If net burdens to the patient from further existence outweigh prospective benefits, the best interests of the patient dictate withholding of medical intervention. Finally, there may be instances when a previously competent and vigorous individual has so deteriorated that the patient's status is so degrading and undignified that a strong majority of people would deem medical intervention to be inhumane. Claire Conroy may well have been one such person.

I reiterate that these principles are applicable in rare and extreme instances. As noted in the discussion of the *Conroy* case, the determination of net benefits and burdens is difficult to make for an incompetent, but conscious patient. With regard to the vast majority of institutionalized individuals, whether persons with mental retardation or senile dementia, it cannot, in good conscience, be said that further existence is not in the best interests of the patient, or that most people would consider the status so degrading and inhumane as to warrant relief.

Artificial administration of nutrition is being increasingly viewed as part of the medical treatment potentially removable according to customary criteria such as substituted judgment and best interests of the patient. This trend is perceptible in cases of permanent coma, or cases such as *Conroy* where the patient is hopelessly ill, i.e., where pathology has set in motion an inexorable dying process.

The question to be faced then becomes whether artificial nourishment is removable from the languishing patient who is not stricken with any immediately life-threatening pathology? That is, if persons are so extremely debilitated that they may be allowed to die upon the onset of a potentially terminal medical condition, can nutrition cessation be viewed as a legitimate approach beforehand—before onset of the life-threatening disease or condition? Is artificial feeding simply a daily medical decision for the severely debilitated population?

The principle that nutrition may sometimes be withheld has been applied only to "artificial" nutrition. The assumption seems universal that if an incompetent patient is physically capable of swallowing and utilizing oral nourishment, such feeding is not classifiable as medical treatment. An alternative view—that nutrition is a form of treatment that need be rendered only when useful to the patient (i.e., when continued existence represents a net benefit)—has not been adopted. In other words, under current standards, manual feeding must always be provided to any patient who continues to accept it. This feeding is deemed part of the palliative or supportive care given to ensure the comfort of languishing, debilitated patients. This category of care includes, besides feeding, analgesics, easing of body position, bowel and bladder management, and provision of a clean and warm environment. The only question mark would be in a hypothetical situation where a patient had, while competent, dictated that he or she not be fed upon reaching the level of disfunction now at hand. Such an instruction with regard to natural feeding is, of course, implausible.

The legal approach is not as clearcut where bodily condition necessitates artificial feeding through medically instituted means even though the patient does not face any other immediately life-threatening condition. This may be the case for some permanent coma victims who, like Karen Ann Quinlan, may subsist for long periods on artificial nutrients without any additional medication. In one recent case involving a ninety-two-year-old (debilitated but not comatose) hospital patient, concurrence of a hiatal hernia and a growth in the patient's esophagus had made a gastrostomy (surgical implantation of a feeding tube in the stomach) the best way of providing nutrition.[30] There was no other acute terminal condition present, but the gastrostomy became an issue because the patient resisted the idea of surgical implantation and had torn out previous feeding tubes. To cite another example, some profoundly retarded individuals may be prone to sucking food into their lungs, causing pneumonia. A surgically implanted tube may then become the only viable means of providing nutrition. In still other instances, gradual deterioration of a patient's faculties may cause an inability to swallow, necessitating artificial feeding. This was part of the picture in the *Conroy* case (though there the patient also faced pathology which was projected to cause death within a year). The trial court there had deemed permanent loss of the swallowing reflex to be reflective of such a vast impairment of brain function as to justify a failure to provide artificial feeding. The appellate courts did not concur in that conclusion. Other patients may retain the swallowing reflex but lose the will to eat. Their refusal to cooperate with manual feeding may then necessitate artificial nourishment.

I suggest that artificial nutrition must be maintained for the languishing patient unless it is found that the previously competent patient would have rejected such medical intervention at this level of disfunction (substituted judgment approach), or unless the presence of physical or emotional suffering makes further existence a net burden to the patient (best interests approach), or unless humane regard for a previously vigorous patient dictates otherwise. Artificial nutrition through an intravenous tube, naso-gastric tube, or gastrostomy constitutes a medical procedure, even though these are also means of providing basic sustenance.[31] Moreover, it is increasingly clear that imminence of death is not necessarily a prerequisite to the removal of life-preserving medical treatment. Karen Ann Quinlan survived nine comatose years purely on intravenous feeding. Yet I have no qualms in asserting, after *Conroy*, that her nourishment was legally removable (if her guardian had so opted) even though *Conroy* spoke solely in terms of removing artificial nourishment from a patient whose projected life span is a year or less.[32] The one year figure is apparently based on the assumption that a natural dying process is then nearing its end. But if a natural dying process has commenced, as would be the case with some conditions prompting artificial nourishment, and if the patient's condition meets the other criteria for permissible withholding of life-prolonging treatment, the one year figure does not seem to furnish a persuasive line.

A more persuasive limitation would be to confine withdrawal of artificial nourishment to situations where the nutrition is associated with an underlying pathology which will inexorably cause the death of the patient. Indeed, this seems to have been the situation in every reported case in which nutrition removal has been authorized (if permanent coma is considered a pathological condition leading to death). This precondition that artificial nutrition be associated with an underlying pathology might differentiate the case of a terribly debilitated mental retardate from a terminally ill cancer patient or victim of a degenerative disease like Alzhemier's disease.

The precondition of underlying terminal pathology might, however, prevent the removal of nutrition from a permanently vegetative patient whose underlying condition (e.g., a ruptured aneurysm) might not be fatal. This does not seem to be a sensible result, as preservation of a permanently vegetative patient seems to serve no benefit to the patient. And, in the case of a previously healthy and vigorous patient, humane consideration might dictate withholding of artificial nutrition. It might be preferable to look at the patient's incapacity to take oral nourishment as part of the underlying pathology. That is, if medical trauma prevents normal feeding (as through a blockage of the esophagus or through brain damage which prevents swallowing), the artificial nourishment becomes part of the medical treatment associated with the pathological condition (such as the brain damage). Then, the patient's condition can be viewed as terminal because he or she would die in the absence of medical intervention. The decision about artificial nourishment can then be made according to the customary criteria—substituted judgment, best interests, or humane consideration.

A contrary approach was recently taken by a trial court judge in Massachusetts who refused to authorize termination of artificial nutrition for a permanently vegetative patient.[33] The patient, forty-eight-year-old Paul Brophy, had been a healthy and vigorous person until, in March of 1983, a ruptured aneurysm caused severe and permanent brain damage. Destruction of brain tissue in the pathways to the cortex left him in a permanently immobile and vegetative state. Mr. Brophy exhibited reflex responses to painful stimuli, but no cognitive function or purposeful interaction with his environment. His nutrition and hydration were sustained via a "G tube," a plastic tube inserted directly into his stomach through an opening which had been surgically created in December 1983. In 1985, when his wife, acting as guardian, sought to have the G tube removed so the patient could be permitted to expire, Mr. Brophy was not facing any major organ disfunction (other than his brain) which would imminently precipitate his death. The medical projection was that he might well survive for several years. (Medical expenses of $10,000 per month were being absorbed by private insurance.)

Mr. Brophy's attending physician and the hospital staff opposed Mrs. Brophy's request to terminate artificial nutrition. Mrs. Brophy then turned to a Massachusetts court to seek official authorization for the proposed removal of the G tube. Justice Kopelman declined to give the authorization even though he found (based on Mr. Brophy's prior statements about terminal care) that the patient would have desired to have the feeding tube removed. The judge was willing to approve a "nonaggressive" treatment strategy under which cardiopulmonary resuscitation would be withheld in the event of heart failure, and antibiotics would be withheld in the event of infection such as bronchitis, but he would not authorize removal of the G tube when death was not otherwise imminent. He ruled that it would be "ethically inappropriate to cause the preventable death of Brophy by the deliberate denial of food and water which can be provided to him in a noninvasive, nonintrusive manner which causes no pain and suffering."[34]

I respectfully suggest that this judicial determination was internally inconsistent and wrong. The *Brophy* court properly did not try to classify the G tube as "nourishment" distinct from medical treatment. Even though the daily administration of substances through the tube might be doable by lay persons, the court acknowledged that the surgical creation of the stomach opening, the formula for nutrition and hydration, and the bimonthly changing of the tube are all essentially medical operations. The court also conceded that even artificial nutrition (such as through a G tube) might be a removable form of medical intervention if death were otherwise imminent.[35] Similarly, while the court purported to stress the noninvasiveness of the daily feeding technique, that factor was not ultimately decisive. For the court conceded both that feeding itself might someday be ceased, and that antibiotics need not be administered if and when an expected bronchial infection were to ensue in the future. Yet administration of antibiotics would not be any more invasive or burdensome to this largely insensate patient than maintenance of the G tube.[36]

Nor did the *Brophy* court contend that cessation of the artificial nutrition would be contrary to Mr. Brophy's "best interests." While the opinion graphically describes the process and effects of starvation and dehydration,[37] there was no contention that the accompanying pain and discomfort would make such a dying process torturous or inhumane. Indeed, Judge Kopelman made an explicit finding that Mr. Brophy would, if competent, order cessation of the G tube. There is no evidence that a person as unaware as Mr. Brophy would suffer at all during a starvation period.

Justice Kopelman appropriately looked to medical ethics for guidance concerning removal of artificial nutrition, but his conclusion seems flawed. True, both the attending physician and the hospital's executive medical committee regarded removal of Mr. Brophy's G tube as "unacceptable and unethical medical practice." But both the Ethics and Disciplinary Committee of the Massachusetts Medical Society (six members) and the Society's General Council (129 members present and voting) adopted resolutions approving removal of artificial nutrition, at least where the patient had previously indicated a wish to discontinue such medical intervention in the condition reached.[38] Despite this strong indication that many physicians would regard removal of Mr. Brophy's G tube as ethically sound, Judge Kopelman enjoined Mrs. Brophy from transferring her husband to another medical facility in order to have the nutrition terminated.

The fact that the patient's vegetative existence was preservable for a protracted period through artificial nutrition was not really determinative. The court was willing to forego other forms of medical treatment—such as antibiotics to fight infection—even though such medical intervention might preserve the patient for a considerable period.[39] In short, none of the court's proclaimed justifications for blocking removal of nutrition—noninvasiveness of the procedure, nonimminence of preventable death, or medical ethics—holds up under scrutiny.

The *Brophy* court refused to look at Mr. Brophy's immediate condition—brain damage sustained because of an aneurysm—as a naturally occurring terminal condition. I disagree. The inability of Mr. Brophy to ingest food was prompted by an aneurysm and its associated brain damage. The surgically implanted and medically maintained artificial nourishment system was no less a product of naturally occurring illness than would be a bronchial infection (as to which antibiotics could, according to the court, be withheld). The same could be said about Mr. Brophy's tracheostomy tube—a tube placed in the trachea to remove excess secretions which could otherwise block the airways. I would treat these last two medical procedures—G tube and tracheostomy tube—in the same manner as the court was willing to treat antibiotic administration or cardiopulmonary resuscitation.

There is an emotional hurdle here, an instinctive revulsion toward cessation of artificial nourishment for patients who would otherwise be sustained for years. To many persons—including Mr. Brophy himself according to his prior expressions—indefinite medical maintenance in a helpless and unaware state represents an even more distasteful spectre. Like permanent coma, persistent vegetative syndrome represents a state in which humane medical handling may well impel a cessation of all forms of medical intervention, including artificial nutrition. I have previously argued that imminence of death should not serve as a precondition to removal of life-preserving medical care, in part because dying patients would needlessly be condemned to prolonged suffering. In the case of insensate, vegetative patients, imposition of an imminence requirement would needlessly condemn such patients to an indefinite, unaware limbo.

The determination of when a chronically ill patient with some level of awareness would be better off dead than alive, so that even simple medical procedures may be omitted, is much more problematical. I suggest that these will be rare cases indeed. Again, with regard to the vast majority of senile or otherwise extremely debilitated persons, it cannot be said that they are better off dead than alive—whether from a perspective of "best interests" of the patient or of "humane" medical handling aimed at respecting human dignity.

As noted above, the incompetent patient's resistance to nutritional efforts is also a factor in determining what best interests or humane handling dictate under the circumstances. That resistance is at least an indication that the artificial nutrition is burdensome in some fashion and distasteful to the patient. If the patient's opposition can be overcome only by lengthy periods of sedation or physical restraint, that fact is relevant in determining whether human dignity (especially in the case of a previously competent patient) demands that medical intervention be foregone.

The same standards applicable to artificial nourishment should apply to "do not resuscitate" (DNR) orders. The main judicial precedent is a 1978 Massachusetts case[40] in which the court upheld entry of a DNR order for a sixty-seven-year-old woman suffering from Alzheimer's disease and from the effects of a massive stroke. She was immobile, speechless, and unaware of her environment. She was sustained by a naso-gastric feeding tube, and her maximum life expectancy was one year. The court, using a substituted judgment approach, found that the patient would not want to be revived to her dismal existence in the event of a cardiac arrest. (No question regarding termination of artificial feeding was raised in the case.)

As in the case of withdrawal of artificial feeding, most DNR orders appear to occur where the patient is terminally ill and death is expected fairly soon.[41] But as the Massachusetts case just mentioned illustrates, death does not have to be imminent in order to justify a DNR order. The national standards for cardiopulmonary resuscitation (CPR) promulgated under the auspices of the AMA also declare that CPR is inappropriate in cases of "terminal irreversible illness."[42] No limit is imposed respecting the projected time span until death. CPR in the face of a terminal, irreversible illness is simply declared a violation of the patient's right to die with dignity.

Under the approach I have suggested above for artificial nourishment (which I would apply as well to DNR decisions), a DNR order would be an option even in the absence of a separate terminal illness. The cardiopulmonary failure would itself constitute a naturally occurring life-threatening process. At that point, decision-makers would have to apply the standards generally applicable to incompetent patients in order to determine whether to administer CPR.

The main controversy surrounding DNR orders appears to relate to decision-making processes rather than criteria. Questions exist about who can initiate such an order, and what procedures must be adhered to in issuing the order. This issue will be examined as part of the next chapter devoted to decision-making processes on behalf of incompetent patients.

V

WHO DECIDES FOR THE INCOMPETENT?

Once a medical patient loses capacity to determine his or her own fate, someone must take responsibility for medical decisions on behalf of the patient. The candidates for surrogate decision-maker are several, each possessing certain positive advantages and carrying certain costs. There is the kindly and learned physician, certainly possessing the maximum knowledge of the patient's medical status and of the range of medical options available. There are the surrounding loved ones, i.e., the next of kin, possessing maximum knowledge of the moribund patient's preferences, tastes, hopes, and aspirations, and presumptively possessing an abiding concern for the patient's welfare. There is an institutional ethics committee, a neutral group capable of assembling diverse views from the fields of medicine, law, and religion and perhaps experienced in facing the intricacies of decisions regarding dying patients. There is the sober and wise judge, capable of gathering and examining all the data relevant to a terminal medical decision, and sensitive to the public interest in protecting innocent life and the sanctity of all human life. There is the trusted friend and confidant of the patient, perhaps designated by the patient himself as the person most attuned to the patient's wishes and most likely to implement what the patient would want done.

Any of these agencies, either singly or in combination, might be appropriate for decision-making on behalf of an incapacitated patient. The normal heavy responsibility for another person's welfare in medical decision-making is, of course, compounded by the life and death nature of the decisions involving moribund patients. Further complicating the picture is the range of medical conditions potentially confronting the decision-maker. Situations range from the patient who has no chance of ever regaining consciousness and facing imminent death to the patient who is potentially salvageable for a considerable period—months or more—and who will be "aware" though not competent to make medical decisions. Another variable is the institutional setting for the particular

105

decision. That setting may run from the sophisticated acute care hospital, to the nursing home or old age home, to the private dwelling. A final variable is the availability or unavailability of persons such as close relatives or friends who can be expected to know the patient's background and preferences, and who can presumptively be trusted to act according to the welfare of the moribund patient.

The current "state of the law" regarding terminal decision-making on behalf of incompetent patients is surprisingly unresolved. The vast majority of states have no legislation specifically covering the issue. More than half the states have statutes which provide for the honoring of "living wills," directives concerning terminal care written while the patient was still competent. But even in those states, no legislative guidance is usually provided regarding incompetent patients who did not previously execute written instructions. Moreover, most of these "living will" statutes specifically preserve the common law rights of patients, thus leaving room for evolution of judicial doctrine.

In practice, the judicial evolution of such doctrine is a gradual process. Medical practices concerning decision-making for incompetent patients develop according to professional mores and perceived exigencies, often without being litigated or otherwise authoritatively examined. Slowly, as cases such as *Quinlan* in New Jersey and *Saikewicz* in Massachusetts arise, the state courts in each jurisdiction are given an opportunity to shape a decision-making process combining one or more of the elements mentioned above. Often, the court limits its determination to the particular kind of case before it, such as that of a comatose patient. Health care providers are then left to improvise solutions for other classes of patients until the judiciary addresses the major types of cases confronting providers.

Each state legislature also has an opportunity to react to the judicially fixed process. But legislative response has been slow, perhaps awaiting guidance from national professional bodies currently engaged in drafting model legislation. In short, development of a definitive and comprehensive legal approach to decision-making authority on behalf of terminally ill, incompetent patients has not yet occurred.

A threshhold issue is whether the courts—as guardians of public norms protecting human life—ought to be directly involved in the actual decision-making process on a regular basis. This would mean judicial examination of the facts of each case and a formal judicial authorization before life-preserving treatment is withdrawn or withheld.

Two of the ground-breaking decisions in the area of incompetent patients, *Quinlan* and *Saikewicz*, appear to take radically different positions regarding judicial involvement in decision-making. They offer a good starting point for a discussion of decision-making processes. *Quinlan* addressed a twenty-two-year-old woman lying in a permanent coma in an acute-care hospital. The court ruled that the woman's natural guardian, her loving father, could serve as the primary decision-maker. This guardian would have to secure the concurrence of an attending physician, the rest of the immediate family, and a hospital ethics committee "or like consultative body" (an idea which will be discussed below). But judicial involvement in the terminal decision was specifically excluded in *Quinlan*. The court declared that judicial intervention would be "a gratuitous encroachment"[1] upon the medical profession's field of competence and would be impossibly cumbersome.

Saikewicz dealt with a sixty-seven-year-old profoundly retarded man facing terminal leukemia in a state institution for the handicapped. The patient had lived in the institution for more than fifty years and his living relatives wanted to have no part in the medical decisions for the patient. The Massachusetts court ruled that only a court could make the ultimate determination whether to withhold chemotherapy from this incompetent patient. According to Judge Liacos' opinion, a judge could and should receive input from a court appointed temporary guardian and from an institutional ethics committee, if one existed, but decision-making authority was to be lodged in a court. A court could, supposedly, best furnish the "detached but passionate investigation and decision" appropriate to such a critical matter. And the court would best reflect the "morality and conscience" of society in reaching a terminal decision.[2]

The Family as Decision-Maker

In caring for incompetent patients, doctors and hospitals have traditionally turned to the patient's next of kin for guidance or instructions in handling a moribund patient.[3] This common practice evolved without explicit endorsement (except by silent acquiescence) from courts and legislatures. A number of considerations have shaped the practice. First, it is assumed that close family members will have the welfare of the patient at heart. Family ties are generally deemed the best instinctive guide to assuring loving solicitude for the incompetent patient. Second, family members are considered best situated to know the wishes, tastes, and preferences of the now incompetent patient. This will enable them to implement the patient's own desires about death and dying, to the extent those desires can be discerned. Third, turning to available family is convenient for the medical personnel and institutions involved. The likely alternative, resort to a court for appointment of a guardian, involves time and bother that the medical personnel would rather dedicate to in-house responsibilities. Hospital staff would prefer to rely on an available source, such as a close family member, rather than devote legal and medical resources to a judicial petition to have a guardian formally appointed to act for the patient. Finally, doctors have enjoyed considerable influence in shaping the ultimate decision when it lay in the hands of next of kin. That is, medical staff have always used their status as information dispensers and respected professionals to exercise suasion in directions preferred by the professionals. Those medical professionals would presumably like to maintain this influence on decision-making.

Allocating terminal decision-making to next of kin or, more realistically, to a concensus of physician and next of kin, is not without certain hazards. Death of a loved one can be a traumatic occasion for the family. There is some concern, then, that confusion, fear, and general emotional upset will interfere with the ability of next of kin to make considered judgments about terminal treatment. In *Quinlan,* for example, the trial judge had qualms about the father of the patient's capacity for dispassionate judgment, even though Mr. Quinlan had always been a loving parent. The judge had therefore appointed an "independent" guardian instead of the father—a decision which the New Jersey Supreme Court overturned. (These elements of emotional involvement probably tend to impel overtreatment rather than neglect.) Another concern is the ultimate objectivity or neutrality of family members. A lingering death can impose emotional and financial strain on the surrounding family. Or the next of kin asked to make decisions may stand to benefit financially from the patient's demise—through inheritance or life insurance proceeds. Some authorities have therefore questioned whether family members are tainted by a potential conflict of interest between their own interests and the well-being of the dying patient.

While the attending physician can be expected to be more dispassionate and objective, even he or she is not 100 percent free from potential distractions. Physicians may be subject to competing interests in the form of institutional resources, other patients demanding attention, and the presence of family anguish. Some physicians may even harbor biases about patients stemming from notions of social utility, socio-economic status, or simply uncooperativeness of the patient.

These spectres of distorted decision-making and even abuse are probably exaggerated. Terminal decisions are not usually made in complete seclusion. The patients are usually institutionalized, within the surveillance of a spectrum of medical personnel and family members. Medical staff are staunchly oriented toward preservation of life, and there is no indication that terminal decisions are lightly undertaken. For a good many years, in a variety of locales, physicians in conjunction with families have withheld or withdrawn life-preserving measures from moribund patients. No pattern of abuse has surfaced.

Nor does the emotional upset of next of kin necessarily preclude their involvement in decision-making. Sensitive input and guidance from medical personnel can ensure that the next of kin understand the medical situation well enough to make an informed judgment despite the trauma accompanying the spectre of death. In situations where the next of kin are too distraught to exercise judgment, or where they are apparently not motivated by concern for the patient, the attending physician and other staff are present as a safeguard. They should be ready to seek appointment of another decision-maker rather than to bow to an ill-considered request from the next of kin.

An alternative arrangement would be to leave decision-making in the hands of the next of kin (in consultation with physicians), only so long as the next of kin have been screened by a court. That is, any next of kin would have to apply to a court to be the formally appointed guardian of the incompetent patient, and the court would screen the good faith and competence of the next of kin before authorizing the appointment. This was the format adopted in 1983 by the Supreme Court of the State of Washington in a case involving termination of treatment to a permanently comatose patient.[4] There, the court, somewhat apprehensive of possible ulterior motives affecting a relative's determinations about terminal treatment, indicated that a judicial designation of the next of kin as guardian would have to precede a termination decision.[5]

The precaution of judicial screening of the next of kin's suitability for terminal decision-making is probably excessive, at least in most of the situations in which a decision to withhold or withdraw life-preserving care is contemplated. (It may be that certain settings, or certain types of decisions, require special procedures, a possibility which will be discussed below.) Ordinarily, hospital personnel should be able to spot decisions reflecting antagonism, insensitivity, or indifference to the interests of the patient. The proper response would then be for the hospital to turn to a court for judicial guidance. In other words, physicians who question the soundness of a relative's choice of treatment or nontreatment for a terminally ill patient should not simply implement the disputed decision. They must either withdraw from the case (if they feel that the course of treatment sought by the next of kin is at least arguably within permissible bounds), or seek judicial appointment of a formal guardian other than the next of kin (if the course of treatment sought seems clearly neglectful of the patient's best interests).

Formal judicial appointment of a guardian would almost inevitably entail expense and delay. As part of a guardianship proceeding, there must be notice to all interested parties (including the patient and all close relatives), there must be a medical report confirming that the patient is indeed incompetent, there must be a hearing at which the potential guardian will have to appear and be cross-examined, and there may have to be a special temporary guardian appointed to present the patient's perspective to the court. Lawyers, including counsel for the hospital, must familiarize themselves with the facts, gather affidavits, and conduct the guardianship hearing. Some postponements may well ensue. In short, the seemingly simple matter of appointment of a guardian will often involve significant delay and expense potentially prolonging and exacerbating the ordeal of both dying patients and their families.

The President's Commission gave extensive consideration to the matter of responsibility for terminal decision-making, and ultimately rejected the idea of automatic judicial screening of the credentials of the next of kin.[6] That body felt that such a guardianship proceeding would be cumbersome and costly in a manner disproportionate to its potential utility. The Commission therefore advised judicial intervention only when the close family cannot agree on a course of conduct, or where the medical personnel view the next of kin's decision as aberrational or unbalanced. That position appears to be well reasoned and sound.

The Commission posited that close family members ordinarily would be concerned with the patient's well-being, and would be sensitive to the patient's previously indicated wishes and preferences. In addition, the Commission regarded family decision-making in this realm as part of the autonomy generally accorded the family as an "important social unit."[7] Finally, the Commission was confident that physicians would exercise an important role in the decision-making process, and would furnish a safeguard against arbitrary decisions by family members. Consequently, the Commission was willing to accord primary decision-making responsibility to family and medical practitioners acting in conjunction.

At the same time, the President's Commission was sensitive both to the ultimate stakes involved—life or death—and the possibilities of error if decision-making were delegated exclusively to family and practitioners. The Commission was therefore receptive to the idea of an institutional review of some or all terminal decisions through the mechanism of an institutional review or "ethics" committee. This, of course, was the mechanism suggested by the *Quinlan* court. That court ruled that a natural guardian's determination on behalf of an incompetent patient would have to be concurred in both by an attending physician and a hospital ethics committee "or like consultative body." The device of an internal committee has therefore drawn some impressive support and deserves examination.

The Institutional Ethics Committee

There is considerable appeal in the idea of an internal committee functioning as part of the decision-making process on behalf of incompetent dying patients. The *Quinlan* court saw such a committee as protective of both patient interests and professional interests by helping to assure that termination decisions are not contaminated by less than worthy motives.[8] That court endorsed the possibility that life and death decision-making might benefit from diffusing responsibility away from a single medical practitioner. The President's Commission also saw merit in a "review" function, arguing that an institutional ethics committee would help ensure that decisions by family and physicians lie "within the range of permissible alternatives."[9] Certainly, such an internal committee offers a mechanism for scrutiny of terminal decisions that is much more expeditious and convenient than judicial appointment of a guardian or actual judicial decision-making (an alternative which will be considered next in this chapter). If the committee is composed of people from diverse disciplines—medicine, law, and religion, for example—there is an opportunity to infuse broad perspectives into the delicate matter of when life-preserving medical treatment can be withdrawn.

The utility of an ethics committee as a guarantor of fair decision-making is by no means established. While the President's Commission felt that the committee device "deserves consideration," their report did not strongly urge implementation of such arrangements. Actual use of ethics committees seems to be growing, but their presence is far from universal in health care institutions. A 1981 survey on behalf of the President's Commission determined that only one percent of all hospitals, and five percent of hospitals with over 200 beds, had already installed such committees.[10] In 1984, there were informal estimates that the number of hospitals which had established ethics committees had grown to ten percent. An informal survey of New Jersey hospitals in 1984 showed that sixty-four percent utilized some form of institutional ethics committee.[11] The state courts have not widely followed *Quinlan*'s lead in mandating involvement of an institutional committee. No recent decision has required an ethics committee to review the substantive decision of physicians and relatives to terminate the treatment of an incompetent dying patient.

Even while there is movement toward voluntarily instituting institutional ethics committees, there is no consensus about how to utilize such a device. Some institutional committees are dominated by medical personnel and their primary function appears to be to confirm the diagnosis and prognosis fixed by the attending physician. Indeed, some such committees are specifically denominated "prognosis committees." Other committees appear to be oriented toward establishing institutional policy and guidelines, but without active involvement in the application of those guidelines to specific cases. Where an ethics committee's function is deemed to include involvement in, or review of, substantive decisions, there is no fixed rule as to whether the committee will function in every case, or whether it will be utilized in particularly difficult decisions. And there is no common approach to the question of whether the committee's function is consultative (advice), decision-making (veto power), or after-the-fact review. Composition of such committees also seems to vary considerably, though a common approach is a multi-disciplinary group including physician, nurse, administrator, lawyer, and clergy.

All of these variables point to the fact that the institutional ethics committee is an institution still very much in its developmental stages, without clear concensus about its composition, function, or even utility. There is suspiciousness of the institution on all sides. Some commentators fear that a committee will diffuse moral responsibility to the extent that immoral decisions will result. Others view such a committee as a meddling, bureaucratic obstacle to sound private decision-making.

The hazards regarding ethics committees would not seem to dictate against their continued use on a trial basis. There may be some danger that such committees would be coopted by the physicians and/or administration of an institution. The result might then be a tendency to rubber stamp professional decisions. Even then there would still be some useful exposure or scrutiny of decisions affecting terminally ill patients. Alternatively, an ethics committeee might turn out to be a cumbersome and/or obstreperous obstacle to sound decision-making by the family in conjunction with the physicians. This would occur, for instance, if a particular committee were dominated by persons believing that every live person must be preserved by all available means, no matter what the patient's prognosis.

But the chances of such a committee existing as a serious hindrance to sound decision-making are not great enough to warrant discarding the idea of ethics committees entirely. In the first place, such committees will not normally be accorded a decision-making or veto power over the full range of terminal decisions. Only when a terminal decision is particularly problematical, as when treatment is sought to be withheld from an incompetent patient who is otherwise preservable for a long period, or when no immediate family or friends are available to guide the medical staff, should a committee's authorization be a precondition to a decision about medical handling. In the remainder of cases, the ethics committee would appear to be a useful device in formulating institutional policy and procedures, in offering guidance when such guidance is sought by physicians or family coping with difficult decisions, and in reviewing some terminal decisions (either when complaints are lodged or on a random basis, or both) to ensure that appropriate guidelines are being followed. Further, even if an internal committee in one institution vetoes a decision reached by physicians and next of kin, an option normally exists of transferring the patient to another institution (so long as the committee in the receiving institution is sympathetic with the proposed course of action).

Courts as Decision-Makers

When the Massachusetts high court assigned ultimate medical decision-making authority over Joseph Saikewicz to a probate court, it sought to promote "detached but passionate investigation and decision."[12] In the abstract, that ideal would indeed be best promoted by judicial involvement in terminal decisions on behalf of incompetent patients. A judge provides a more "impartial" decision-maker than either family members potentially influenced by financial considerations or their own suffering or discomfort, or doctors potentially distracted by the needs of the institution or other patients or the family's anguish. Legal procedures of subpoena of witnesses, and of examination and cross-examination under oath offer a more exhaustive and careful information gathering process than the informal efforts of family and hospital staff (even if aided by an ethics committee). Participation of a judge also tends to ensure sensitivity to the emerging legal standards of decision-making (substituted judgment, best interests, etc.), along with careful application of the particular facts to the prevailing legal norms. Moreover, as judges continue to analyze various circumstances, and draft reasoned explanations for their decisions, development of a body of guiding principles is promoted. The public exposure provided in judicial examination of the emerging principles, and their application to specific cases, helps ensure that emerging practices conform to societal norms. Such public exposure also serves, of course, as a preventive against any possible abuse of helpless incompetent patients.

Despite these attractions of a judicial role in decision-making, it is becoming increasingly clear that regularized judicial participation in terminal decisions is neither practical nor desirable. Even if judicial proceedings in terminal cases are handled on an expedited basis, the prospects are strong for a time consuming, costly, and burdensome process. Lawyers must be involved to represent the interests of the institution, the family, the patient (a special guardian is commonly appointed), and sometimes even the state (in the form of the local prosecutor). All these lawyers participate in fact gathering through presentation and examination of witnesses. Physicians and family are called to testify. Postponements to accommodate the various schedules involved are almost inevitable. If the trial court renders a prompt decision, there is still a possibility of an appeal with attendant delays and accumulating costs.

The net result is that judicial involvement tends to be cumbersome and expensive. Conscientious family and hospital staff may well be deterred from making appropriate terminal decisions. For neither relatives nor doctors wish to undertake the time, effort, and expense involved. The public exposure accompanying judicial proceedings does more than ensure the neutral scrutiny of a judge. It exposes a normally delicate and anguishing decision to the glare of potential publicity and reaction from extremists who would automatically oppose any termination of human life. To the extent there is either deterrence or delay of appropriate decisions, the consequence is to "prolong the physical suffering of the patient and aggravate the distress of a family already confronting the emotional and financial pressures of coping with a serious illness."[13] In several of the reported cases in which litigation was involved, the patient languished and ultimately died before a final judicial decision on termination of treatment could be obtained.[14] The delay usually extended over several months and sometimes for more than a year.

The perceptible trend among courts, legislatures, and commentators alike is to avoid regularized judicial involvement in the numerous situations in which withholding or withdrawing of life-preserving care to an incompetent patient is considered. Courts in California, Florida, Georgia, Minnesota, and Washington have indicated, between 1983 and 1985, that at least certain types of termination decisions can be made by family and physicians without judicial involvement in the actual decision-making process. All these rulings recognize that judicial participation can be cumbersome and disruptive of the large number of decisions that must inevitably be faced. They all recognize that judicial review is available if any interested party raises objections about the substance of a particular decision.

While abjuring direct judicial participation in initial decision-making, these recent decisions have not allocated unfettered authority to the next of kin and physicians acting in conjunction. In one instance, a court looked to participation of an institutional ethics committee as a helpful safeguard in the decision-making process,[15] and in another instance a court dictated involvement of a prognosis review committee.[16] But only in two instances, both without extensive consideration of the appropriate decision-making process, have courts outside of Massachusetts shown willingness to actively participate in decisions whether to terminate life-preserving treatment for an incompetent adult patient.[17] The recent judicial trend is clearly away from regularized involvement in such decisions.

In the few states in which legislatures have addressed the question of surrogate decision-making for incompetent dying patients, the tendency is also to avoid judicial involvement in the actual decision-making process. Recent statutes in Arkansas, Florida, New Mexico, North Carolina, Louisiana, Oregon, and Virginia all permit terminal decisions to be made by physicians and next of kin operating in conjunction with one another, but without direct judicial involvement.[18] While these statutes allow private decision-making, they do limit the circumstances in which a termination decision can be made. For example, in Virginia the terminal decision by family and physician is confined to situations where the patient is in an irreversibly terminal condition and death is imminent.[19] And in North Carolina and Oregon, the only explicit legislative authorization of termination of an incompetent patient's life-preserving treatment is for a permanently comatose patient.[20]

Such statutes as those in Virginia and Oregon authorize terminal decisions on narrower grounds than the judicially developed standards described earlier. They thus pose more of a hindrance than a help. Physicians may be deterred from implementing sound and humane decisions because the patient's condition does not fall within the class of terminal decisions specifically endorsed by the legislature.

The bulk of legal commentary favors the trend away from regularized judicial involvement in decisions to withhold or withdraw life-preserving treatment from incompetent adults. The President's Commission, under the tutelage of law professor Alexander Capron, concluded that regular judicial intervention would be "unduly intrusive, slow, and costly and would frame treatment decisions in misleadingly adversarial terms."[21] Another searching examination of decision-making procedures, published in 1984, also argued that the judicial role should be confined to review of the occasional private decision alleged to deviate from acceptable norms. That study concluded:

> For most right to die decisions, courts should not be the place of either first or last report. Routine involvement of the judicial process . . . [in decisions for critically ill adults] is not warranted by logic or experience.[22]

Student law review commentary also supports the notion that a courtroom is not the appropriate forum for the bulk of treatment decisions involving incompetent dying patients.[23]

To withhold a regular judicial role in decision-making is not to forego all judicial scrutiny of the delicate matter of when life-preserving treatment may be withdrawn from incompetent patients. Even if a court is not made the primary decision-maker, indirect judicial involvement will generally be available. No matter who is authorized to make an initial terminal decision, judicial review of the processes and criteria can be expected when next of kin seek to compel an uncooperating institution to comply with their wishes to terminate care, or where the institution seeks judicial appointment of a special guardian on the basis that the natural guardian has refused to set a proper treatment course. Occasionally, judicial review may also ensue through criminal prosecutions, or malpractice claims, or review of professional disciplinary proceedings. Such judicial review would not take place on a regular or routine basis, but would occur where interested persons—relatives of the patient, friends, or hospital staff, for example—press claims of abuse of acceptable norms of decision-making. Another possible form of indirect judicial involvement in decision-making would be judicial appointment of the agent or guardian authorized to make any termination determination, with accompanying scrutiny of the good faith and competence of the potential guardian.

Even in Massachusetts, where *Saikewicz* had been viewed as requiring judicial participation in terminal decisions regarding incompetents, the drift is away from regularized judicial involvement. After *Saikewicz*, there was a considerable outcry in the Massachusetts medical community about the potential disruption of ongoing medical processes surrounding terminally ill patients. The author of the *Saikewicz* opinion, Justice Paul Liacos, responded in an article that the decision had been misread. He explained that the court's intention had been to involve the judiciary only "from time to time" as a safeguard in particular decisions "fraught with difficulties."[24] And sure enough, in a 1980 decision called *In re Spring*,[25] the Supreme Judicial Court of Massachusetts indicated that a number of factors would determine whether judicial examination of a termination decision is required. Among the factors cited were: whether the patient is housed in a state institution; whether there is a family member present ostensibly operating in good faith; the patient's prognosis; and the clarity of professional opinion in the case.[26] The import of the post-*Saikewicz* decisions in Massachusetts appears to be that judicial review of a nontreatment determination is not required where treatment would at most produce only a brief extension of life, and a caring family is present to guide the doctors.

The Massachusetts experience tends to confirm that no procedural approach should be applied across the board to all incompetent patients. It is becoming possible to classify cases which can be left to private channels, and to identify other classes of cases in which special scrutiny may be warranted. The next subsection treats the emerging need for variable processes based on the medical status of the patient involved.

Variable Procedures According to Prognosis of the Patient

With Massachusetts' retreat from the broad implications of *Saikewicz,* the pronounced trend is away from regularized judicial involvement in termination decisions involving incompetent adults. The challenge now is to define classes of cases in which decision-making principles are well established, and in which such principles are routinely applied to actual cases without reported abuse. Those decisions can safely be left to the traditional decision-making processes—medical staff and next of kin acting in conjunction with one another.

The clearest case of permissible termination which has emerged in the years of discussion since *Quinlan* is that of the permanently comatose patient. Judicial decisions now establish both that permanent coma is medically identifiable with fair certainty, and that no meaningful gain inures to a patient prolonged in such an indefinite limbo. These principles having been uniformly accepted, there would appear to be no reason not to allow family and physicians to terminate life-preserving care for a permanently comatose patient, or for a noncomatose patient locked in a persistent vegetative state without consciousness.

In fact, there is a perceptible judicial trend in the direction of placing such decisions in the hands of family and physicians. *Quinlan,* operating as a ground-breaker, included an ethics committee "or like consultative body" as a part of the decision-making machinery. Only one other decision (in Minnesota) has endorsed participation by an ethics committee in a decision to remove treatment from a patient in a permanent coma.[27] One court (in Washington State) has required concurrence of a "prognosis committee"—i.e., medical confirmation of the comatose condition of the patient.[28] Three courts have indicated that the next of kin and physicians can withdraw life-support from a permanently comatose patient without an ethics committee and without judicial approval of the decision.[29]

I suggest that a recent Florida decision in *John F. Kennedy Memorial Hospital v. Bludworth*,[30] sets a pattern which will eventually be replicated elsewhere. In speaking to the case of a patient diagnosed as permanently comatose, the Florida Supreme Court rejected the necessity of either a hospital ethics committee or judicial scrutiny. The sole outside element injected in the process was a requirement that two medical specialists confirm that the patient is in a permanently vegetative status. Otherwise, the terminal decision can be relegated to traditional private channels. The court commented:

> The decision to terminate artificial life supports [to a permanently co-matose patient] is a decision that normally should be made in the patient-doctor-family relationship. Doctors, in consultation with close family members, are in the best position to make these decisions.[31]

This process, in which decisions regarding a permanently comatose patient are relegated to the attending physician and next of kin, with expert medical consultation, seems highly appropriate to the class of patients involved.

Another class of patients for whom decisions can safely be allocated to the immediate family and attending physician is that of incompetent terminal patients whose demise is both unavoidable and imminent. No source wants to define imminence for this purpose, and I'm no braver than the rest. But the typical approach is to speak in terms of days, or a few weeks, and not months. When an incompetent dying patient has reached this stage, it is common to speak of medical intervention as prolonging the dying process rather than preserving life. The basic medical object becomes to ease that dying process for the patient and to keep the patient as comfortable as possible. Thousands upon thousands of decisions about withholding one form or another of medical intervention are made each year on behalf of such waning patients.

The prevailing decision-making format for such hopelessly ill patients is through immediate family or next of kin in conjunction with medical personnel. As early as 1973, the American Medical Association went on record in favor of allowing the immediate family to dictate withholding of certain medical procedures for an incompetent patient whose death is imminent. Recent reports in medical journals confirm that this approach has become prevalent—that physicians in conjunction with next of kin frequently withhold some forms of life-preserving treatment from incompetent patients who are "clearly in the terminal phase of an irreversible illness."[32] These practices are so widespread, and the absence of abuse so reassuring, that it is unlikely that decision-making in this class of cases will be altered by judicial or legislative tampering. In fact, some of the fledgling legislative efforts regarding surrogate decision-making appear to endorse rather than disrupt such ongoing practices.[33] Judicial tribunals can be expected to follow suit and approve the existing decision-making pattern in the rare instances when such decisions reach litigation.

The really problematic cases are those in which an incompetent, terminally ill patient is aware in some fashion and salvageable, with treatment, for a period of months or more. Especially if the patient was never competent, like Joseph Saikewicz (the profoundly retarded sixty-seven-year-old suffering from terminal leukemia), determining "best interests" or "humane treatment" is a Solomonian task. A life-prolonging option always exists in such cases, but must be considered in light of the burden which continued existence entails for the incompetent patient. In such instances, some scrutiny of a termination decision reached by family and doctors may be called for. The legal norms are still evolving in this class of cases, and there is a societal interest in ensuring that these terminal decisions are reviewed by some source outside the narrow confines of the family-doctor relationship.

As noted above, an institutional ethics committee offers a possible safeguard without implicating the burdensome judicial process. It would be appropriate to require consultation with the ethics committee without affording that committee a veto power. In the event that the ethics committee regards a proposed decision (jointly made by next of kin and physicians) as outside acceptable bounds, the institution can seek judicial appointment of an official guardian (other than the next of kin). Judicial review of the allegedly aberrational decision would then be forthcoming.

There may be other variables—beside the prognosis of the dying patient—which should bear on the decision-making machinery employed to determine the incompetent patient's medical treatment. The institutional setting, and the absence of close relatives or friends surrounding the moribund patient, may be other relevant factors. The discussion in this chapter has basically assumed that the patient is located in a hospital, and that there is an available next of kin to participate in decision-making. But critical medical decisions may be faced in a variety of institutional settings—including state institutions for the handicapped, and private nursing homes—and with total absence of interested or caring relatives.

Conditions in many public institutions for the mentally handicapped are notoriously problematical for purposes of medical decision-making. These institutions are commonly understaffed, and the patient population is sometimes burdensome if not outright disruptive. Because of low salary scales, the professional staff that is attracted may tend to be of a lesser calibre than the average personnel outside of such institutions. In terms of medication, there has been a strong tendency to overuse behavior regulating drugs in order to minimize management problems with the incompetent patients.[34] Many of the patients are isolated from the outside world, without caring relatives or friends to help safeguard patient interests.

In the absence of close relatives or a formal guardian, medical staff in such institutions have tended to use their own best judgment in making medical decisions for incompetent patients. Such an arrangement for life-preserving treatment decisions would appear to be unacceptable. Such decisions are too insulated from scrutiny, and the temptations of ulterior motivation too natural, to allow medical personnel an unfettered discretion. Some autonomous agency, such as an ombudsman or other agency charged with representing patient interests, should be privy to any terminal decisions in such a setting, with an option to turn to a judicial or administrative body in the event of disagreement with the attending physician about the wisdom of any particular medical determination. That is, house staff should be required to obtain concurrence from a person or agency independent of institutional control before implementing any decision removing life-preserving treatment from an institutionalized, incompetent patient. Where an ostensibly caring relative is part of the decision-making process, this outside scrutiny might be dispensed with so long as the case falls into one of the categories described above—permanent lack of cognition or imminent demise.

Nursing homes present another setting in which some patients are both handicapped (by impaired mental functioning) in coping with medical decisions, and isolated from a family support framework. In the recent *Conroy* decision dealing with terminal care for an eighty-four-year-old barely conscious resident of a private nursing home, the New Jersey Supreme Court expressed grave reservations about leaving terminal decisions in the nursing home context to the normal internal processes involving medical staff and next of kin, if present. Despite the presence of a loving nephew willing to guide medical decisions on behalf of Ms. Conroy, the court dictated a fairly complex decision-making procedure. The key elements were that judicial review must be obtained of the next of kin's credentials to act as guardian with authority to request removal of life-preserving treatment, and that a state ombudsman must investigate the case and give approval before any termination of treatment. An attending physician, and the rest of the family would also have to concur. Finally, medical confirmation of the patient's prognosis was also required.

The New Jersey Supreme Court's concerns about the fair treatment of nursing home populations are readily understandable. But the solution imposed may be too extreme. Especially where there is a concerned relative operating in ostensible good faith, the need for costly and time-consuming judicial examination of the potential guardian's good faith would appear to be unnecessary.[35] Next of kin would seem to be motivated by the same considerations as would be present if the patient were housed in a hospital, and no judicial screening of a next of kin's bona fides would take place, under *Quinlan*, if the patient were in a hospital rather than a nursing home. Presence of an ombudsman should serve as a sufficient safeguard against abuse of patients' interests. Moreover, if there is a conscientious next of kin available, and if the patient falls within one of the classes of cases mentioned above—i.e., is permanently lacking cognition or is facing imminent death—even the ombudsman's involvement would appear to be excessive.

If there is no next of kin to act for the nursing home patient, then scrutiny by an ombudsman or an institutional ethics committee would seem appropriate regardless of the prognosis class into which the patient might fall. Otherwise, a physician would be making virtually unexamined decisions about a waning patient. *Conroy* eschewed an ethics committee on the basis that nursing homes, as modest sized institutions compared to hospitals, would not readily be able to organize such committees. New Jersey happened to have had in place an administrative office (ombudsman) specifically charged with surveillance of nursing home operation. Resorting to that agency as a watchdog of nursing home termination decisions was therefore natural. Other jurisdictions might prefer to use some version of an institutional ethics committee to diffuse responsibility away from the sole hands of an attending physician, at least where a nursing home patient has no close family member or friend willing to share in medical decision-making.[36] The same technique could be employed even where an ostensibly conscientious next of kin is present, but the dying patient has some level of awareness and is potentially salvageable for months or longer. Such decisions are so delicate that involvement beyond the family-physician circle may indeed be appropriate.

Patient's Appointment of a Proxy Decision-Maker

A philosophy professor at Brown University recently wrote:

> The prospect of life-terminating decisions being made by doctors (whose values may be completely different from the patient's) or family members (who often have vested emotional and financial interests in the patient's prompt demise) is enough to frighten anyone with the temerity to value his own life.[37]

Anyone this wary of having terminal decisions made through the normal decision-making channels described above might well consider appointment of a trusted person to make critical medical decisions in the event the appointor becomes incompetent. In fact, there are distinct advantages to a patient-designated proxy which make the system broadly appealing whether a person is wary of doctors and/or family or not.

The assumption behind a designated proxy is that the designator will not only choose a particularly dependable person to act as surrogate decision-maker, but that extensive conversations will be held instructing the proxy about the wishes and preferences of the designator. If this assumption is fulfilled, the advantages of the designated proxy are patent. A specific individual then exists at the moment of critical decision-making who is intimately familiar with the now incompetent patient's wishes. This eases the tasks of medical staff both by providing important information in the fact gathering process regarding the patient's previously expressed wishes, and by avoiding confusion about legal authority such as occurs when close family are not available or are not unanimous in their desires. Moreover, the proxy furnishes someone to act as an advocate of the patient's position and potential enforcer of the patient's wishes, should medical staff be reluctant to follow the patient's previously expressed desires.

The proxy is a better informed decision-maker than the patient who speaks through a living will. That is, the drafter of a living will usually must attempt to anticipate the prospective circumstances surrounding the dying process. This speculation may come well in advance of the actual decline and incompetency. It is difficult to foresee and deal with the multitude of relevant variables and their permutations. The proxy, by contrast, possesses full information about the patient's condition and the treatment options at the very moment of decision-making.

The system may not be foolproof. There is nothing to guarantee that a proxy will be available at the critical locale at the critical moment, or that the proxy won't waver in his resolve to fulfill the patient's wishes. A patient's prior revocation of a proxy appointment might go unnoticed. There is even some chance that medical personnel might prematurely turn to a proxy for instructions before a waning patient has really lost competency.[38] Or wrangling and confusion may ensue when next of kin (if not designated as the proxy) object either to the fact that someone else is charged with decision-making authority, or to the substance of the proxy's decision. But these speculative problems would not seem to detract from the overall utility of a designated proxy in the decision-making process for an incompetent dying patient.

The legal effectiveness of a proxy designation is not fully established. Only three states (Delaware, California, and Virginia) statutorily authorize the appointment of an agent for purposes of medical decision-making. In the absence of statute, traditional common law doctrine holds that some decisions are too intimate to be effectively delegated to an agent; thus common law doctrine poses a potential barrier to legal enforcement of a proxy appointment for terminal medical decisions. Chances are very good that a simple document known as a "durable power of attorney" will be recognized as an effective instrument allowing a person to designate a surrogate to make critical medical decisions should the patient become incompetent.[39] The power of attorney is a writing conferring upon a person authority to perform specified actions on behalf of the signer. Durable refers to the continuation of the document's effect after the incapacity of the signer.

With the strong trend of judicial opinion toward recognition of autonomy and self-determination in shaping the dying process, the prospects are good for acceptance of a durable power of attorney or similar appointment of a surrogate decision-maker. The *Conroy* court, in dictum, expressed willingness to uphold appointment of a proxy.[40] No court has expressed principled opposition to the idea. Because the proxy is such a simple device, yet offers some reassurance that a person's concerns about a prospective dying process will be honored, it may become the wave of the future in decision-making for incompetent patients.

VI

DEFECTIVE INFANTS

Approximately four percent of births in the United States involve some form of congenital abnormality. The range of such abnormalities is, of course, vast—from minor correctible defects, to serious permanent handicaps, to irreversibly fatal conditions.[1] An extreme example is the anencephalic infant born with total or almost total absence of a brain. Such an infant is fated to die within a short period regardless of medical intervention. But partial anencephalics, those with no forebrain or mid-brain, could potentially be preserved for lengthy periods, though limited to primitive functioning barely characteristic of human life.

There are numerous serious birth anomalies less extreme than the total absence of brain tissue. For example, infants born at very low weight—below 1500 grams—commonly face serious heart and/or lung impairments. Amazing techniques—including intricate respirators, sensitive monitoring devices, and other mechanical wonders—have been developed to deal with and salvage infants with underdeveloped lungs or other organs. Despite these sophisticated techniques, many low birth weight infants will eventually succumb, sometimes after a prolonged and torturous struggle. On occasion, survival is obtained, but at a serious price. Vigorous medical intervention may itself produce negative side effects (known as iatrogenic conditions) such as blindness, brain damage, or cerebral palsy.[2]

In addition, there are a variety of chromosomal deficiencies with which infants are sometimes born. Trisomy 21, or Down's syndrome, is probably the best known. This condition, often accompanied by a heart defect, results in a range of I.Q.'s between twenty-five and sixty—in other words, in various degrees of serious mental retardation. With vigorous medical intervention, however, the life expectancy of the typical Down's infant is forty to sixty years. Other chromosomal deficiencies are more lethal. For example, trisomy 18, occurring once in 3500 live births, is fatal in ninety percent of the cases within one year. Those infants surviving the first year typically face serious brain abnormalities, congenital heart disease, respiratory tract problems, gastrointestinal and liver deformities, and little chance of living beyond their second birth-day. Trisomy 13 produces severe mental retardation along with blind-ness, deafness, heart defects, and deformities of limbs. Survival can be maintained with respirators, pacemakers, catheters, and other medical intervention, but the existence salvaged is severely impaired.

A variety of neurological disorders are also confronted in neonatal care units. Spina bifida cystica presents a common (one out of 1000 live births) and perplexing situation.[3] The condition involves a defect in the structure of the spinal cord with the result that part of the cord pro-trudes from the infant's back. Depending on the level of the lesion and other factors, the accompanying disabilities vary in severity. In the most severe cases, consequences of spina bifida include paralysis of the limbs, incontinence of the bowel and bladder, and severe mental retardation. In the middle range of spina bifida, the prospects are partial paralysis (with possible mobility via braces or crutches), incontinence, a shunt (to drain excess fluid from the brain) in order to cope with the hydro-cephalus frequently found, and a thirty percent chance of some mental retardation. All spina bifida survivors will require multidisciplinary man-agement—neurosurgeons, urologists, orthopedists, physiotherapists, nurses, and social workers—for indefinite periods of time.

Without surgery, ninety-eight percent of spina bifida infants die. The vast majority of that group die within one year, but six percent in one study survived untreated for more than two years.[4] For those untreated patients who survive, their condition is poorer than if they had been treated; complications include hydrocephalus, cortical blindness, and kyphosis (extreme curvature of the spine). With surgery to close the lesion and to install a shunt (where hydrocephalus is present), the sur-vival rate is much higher, approximately seventy percent. The surgical interventions themselves carry a five percent risk of death and, on occasion, may risk exacerbating the degree of paralysis. (Without sur-gery, the chances of death are clearly much higher.) Medical strategies toward spina bifida infants have fluctuated over the years. Currently, with improved techniques of shunting, catheterization, and neonatology generally, the trend among physicians is toward recommending medical intervention for most but not all infants afflicted with the condition.

Other neurological conditions are invariably fatal. For example, Tay-Sachs disease, which appears when a child is six to nine months old, is fatal by age five. In the meantime, the disorder results in blindness and gradual deterioration of motor function and mentation until an insen-sate existence is reached in the last stage before death.

This spectrum of conditions and impairments presents anguishing dilemmas to those charged with medical decisions regarding defective infants. The initial question is whether to undertake full medical and surgical intervention in order to preserve the maximum life span of the stricken infant. In the case of a very premature infant with under-developed lungs, the question may be whether to administer oxygen therapy. For a Down's syndrome infant with an atresia (blockage) preventing normal nutrition and digestion, the question is whether to perform surgery to remove the blockage. For the spina bifida cystica case, the issue may be whether to operate to close the back lesion, or whether to install a shunt to ease the consequences of hydrocephalus, where present.

The considerations which come into play are numerous. If medical intervention is omitted or diminished in intensity, what will be the status of the infant? Will death ensue and, if so, after what period and with what consequences to the infant during the dying process? If death will not ensue in the short term, what will be the infant's condition (degree of affliction and handicap in the longterm)? If full medical intervention is undertaken, what will the likely impact be on the infant? What are the chances of saving the infant's life? What degree of disfunction or handicap will result despite medical intervention? What amount of physical pain and/or emotional suffering will the child undergo both in the short and long terms as a result of vigorous treatment? What alternative forms of medical treatment are available? What will the impact be on the parents and siblings from raising a handicapped child? What alternatives to home care are available? How much will medical treatment cost and who will be responsible for those expenses?

The medical decision-maker must also cope with issues relating to the legal bounds applicable to handling newborns. Under what circumstances do the legal strictures of homicide, malpractice, and/or child neglect permit the withholding of life-preserving medical treatment from a defective infant? What legal standard governs such a terminal decision? Can the interests of parents and siblings be considered in reaching such a terminal decision? Can the potential economic burdens on the family or on society be considered? Indeed, who possesses the ultimate decision-making authority? The attending physician? The parents? A hospital committee? A court?

These law related issues will be discussed below. As an introduction, it is important to note that the law is in a state of flux and definitive answers are not available. The relatively few judicial expressions on point are found in lower court decisions which don't have widespread binding effect. There is no pathfinding precedent by a high level court such as occurred with the *Quinlan* decision in New Jersey.

Some movement toward legislative intervention in medical handling of defective newborns is discernible. Federal involvement has taken two forms—first, federal regulations pursuant to the federal statute relating to discrimination against the handicapped and, second, federal regulations pursuant to 1984 amendments to the federal statute governing grants to states for programs to combat child abuse. Those 1984 amendments require participating states (those applying for and receiving federal grants) to conform their child abuse prevention measures to a federal definition of child abuse which includes nontreatment of some defective newborns. Several recent state laws are also intended to regulate practices in the neonatal wards of hospitals. But, as will emerge from the discussion below, the precise meaning and effect of all such laws is as yet undetermined. The legislative developments will be examined later.

That the law relevant to defective infants is in flux emerges from an overview of the lower court decisions which have spoken to the issue up till now. Before 1982, the clear tendency of courts was to intervene and to order life-preserving treatment for defective infants whose parents opposed such treatment.[5] In at least three recorded instances, judges ordered surgical treatment for infants suffering from spina bifida. In one of those instances, the child's lesion was low; consequently, the prognosis was that the child would be able to walk with braces, and would enjoy normal intellectual development. The New York court noted in its order (grounded on the child neglect statute) that the child had "a reasonable chance to live a useful, fulfilled life."[6]

That was New York in 1979. In Maine, in 1974, surgical intervention to implant a feeding tube was judicially ordered even though the prognosis was that the spina bifida baby would be blind, deaf, palsied, and might never gain full consciousness. A local judge overruled the parents' objections and commented:

> Parents have no right to withhold such treatment and . . . to do so constitutes neglect in the legal sense. The basic right enjoyed by every human being is the right to life itself.[7]

More recently, in Florida in 1981, a local court directed surgery for a spina bifida infant despite the parents' reliance on medical advice from two of four examining physicians that treatment should be omitted.[8]

Similarly, a number of lower courts have intervened to order surgery for mongoloid (Down's syndrome) infants with correctable feeding blockages (atresia).[9] In another instance, a Massachusetts judge directed surgery for a month old infant suffering numerous impairments from congenital rubella, including cataracts on both eyes, deafness, congenital heart failure, respiratory difficulties, and severe retardation. The judge there voiced a determination to save the infant's life "regardless of the quality of that life."[10]

This judicial disposition to regard any newborn life, even one severely handicapped, as preferable to no life at all, and hence a judicial willingness to prevent withholding of life-preserving treatment, seems to have been modified since 1982. That year, a Massachusetts court approved entry of a no code (do not resuscitate) order for a four and one-half month old infant with cyanotic heart disease and associated lung problems.[11] Because of an uncorrectable blood flow deficiency, the infant was fated to die within a year.

A Florida court in 1984 upheld the removal of life support systems from a ten month old infant who had been born with severe brain damage and who would never emerge from a "permanent vegetative coma."[12] In the most controversial case yet, in which a court refused to override a decision to withhold life-preserving care from a defective infant, Indiana courts in 1982 allowed a mongoloid infant to die of starvation without surgery needed to correct a blockage and anomaly in the infant's digestive tract.[13] This was known as the Baby Doe or Infant Doe case and provoked a series of federal regulations, to be discussed below, aimed at compelling life-preserving treatment for most defective newborns.

This recent judicial trend—to acknowledge that there are some situations in which life-preserving medical treatment may legitimately be withheld from defective infants—begins to move the courts closer to what appears to have been common medical practice for some time. Certainly, there are a number of anecdotal reports of necessary surgery and/or feeding being withheld from mongoloid children.[14] In those instances, no judicial intervention was sought and the infants were permitted to die. Another index of medical attitudes is a 1976 survey of 276 pediatric surgeons belonging to the American Academy of Pediatrics. That survey disclosed that seventy-seven percent of these surgeons would acquiesce in a parental determination not to clear a feeding blockage from a Down's syndrome infant.[15] In that same survey, it emerged that eighty-three percent of the surgeons did not believe it was necessary to try and provide life-preserving treatment for all salvageable infants, and sixty percent of them would acquiesce in a decision not to perform surgery in a spina bifida case.

These figures reflect a widespread medical attitude that it is not appropriate to employ medical advances in neonatology to preserve every newborn, no matter how impaired the prospective existence. Selective treatment has been an apparent watchword for some time. At one time, that approach may have been primarily employed in the rare case of an infant "monster"—a newborn so grossly malformed that its human qualities are obscured. But by 1973 Doctors Duff and Campbell reported that fourteen percent of infant deaths ($^{43}/_{299}$) occurring at Yale New Haven Hospital between January 1970 and June 1972 were associated with considered decisions to withhold medical treatment from infants afflicted with various impairments.[16] It was also in the early 1970's that public debate emerged about selecting which infants suffering from spina bifida cystica should receive aggressive medical treatment.[17] (The remainder would be provided supportive care to ease the dying process.)

In short, there appears to have been a sharp divergence between medical practices and the view expressed by some lower court judges, described above, that failure to provide life-preserving treatment to a defective newborn constitutes child neglect. Before attempting to resolve whether and when life-preserving care may legally be withheld from a defective infant, it may be helpful to resolve who is authorized to make critical medical determinations for a helpless newborn.

Decision-Making for Defective Infants

Traditionally, a decision whether to provide life-preserving care for a defective infant often devolved upon the attending physician or physicians. Sometimes, this may have been by default of the parents, either because they were intimidated by the institutional setting or befuddled by the complexity of the underlying issues. But many doctors believed and continue to believe that medical personnel are in principle best situated to make the critical medical decisions regarding a defective infant's fate. Their assumption is that physicians possess both the expertise and detached judgment needed to make a considered determination about the complex issue. The 1976 national survey of pediatricians, referred to above, indicated that thirty-three percent of pediatricians and pediatric surgeons surveyed felt that attending physicians should carry "the major reponsibility" for any decision to allow a severely impaired infant to die.[18] The same attitude—that a physician should be the primary decision-maker—is reflected in a number of articles by medical authorities on the subject of handling defective newborns.[19]

Despite this assertion of authority by many physicians, the trend is clearly away from leaving primary responsibility for these matters in the hands of attending physicians. Recognition is now widespread that a decision about life-preserving treatment for a defective infant is not exclusively a medical issue. Accurate medical prognosis is one critical element in decision-making, but the medical facts must be processed and assessed in light of all the circumstances and interests of the infant. (The precise standards for decision-making will be discussed later.) Law, ethics, and social values all come into play. As to these latter issues, a physician's expertise is no greater than that of many other persons.

As public debate grows about the handling of defective newborns, the medical community generally seems to be withdrawing from any assertion of dominion over these life and death treatment determinations. The American Academy of Pediatrics, in a statement issued in October of 1983, recommended a thorough review of each decision not to continue critical treatment.[20] This apparently was intended to mean not only close conferral with parents, but consultation with legal, ethical, and medical experts, and possibly with a "bioethics review committee." The American Medical Association's Judicial Council has gone even further and suggested that any decision to terminate an infant's life-preserving treatment is the choice of parents.[21] Thus, major organizations representing physicians have disclaimed any notion that physicians should be allocated exclusive decision-making authority for these thorny decisions. Of course, the attending physician—as the primary source of information and input about the infant's status and prospects—will almost inevitably exercise considerable influence on decision-making no matter where the official authority lies.

Under the current legal framework, decision-making responsibility lies in the hands of the infant's parents in consultation with medical staff.[22] This is true even though a decision to decline medical intervention may effectively mean the death of the infant. There are several explanations. First, the vast majority of decisions involving minors in a family unit are customarily left in the hands of the adult family members free of government interference in the decision-making process. This tradition of family autonomy is a venerable one in the United States. Government intervention is generally confined to fixing the bounds of permissible decisions and intervening in the case of aberrational decisions. The initial decision on care of a child is conferred on the parents.

Another factor is the underlying assumption that by and large parents operate with the best interests of their bodily issue at heart—that parental ties of affection and responsibility will generally prompt decisions sensitive to the needs of children. No confidence exists that any combination of judicial or administrative decision-makers would produce better decisions, even if some arrangement for nonparental decision-making were administratively feasible. Finally, there is some inclination to allocate decisions about an infant's fate to those who will likely bear the burdens of the potential outcome. The assumption is that parents will be impacted strongly by raising a severely impaired child in the event that a decision for aggressive medical intervention is reached.

Many medical and legal commentators have criticized application of this traditional framework of parental prerogatives to the context of life and death decisions for defective infants. These authorities question whether parents of defective newborns have the capacity to make careful, considered judgments in this context. The principal claim is that parents will likely be "emotionally and cognitively overwhelmed and exhausted" at the critical point in time.[23] Psychological data is cited to the effect that parents of such infants are initially overwrought and assailed by reactions such as "numbness, grief, disgust, rage, [or] disbelief" prompting a negative attitude toward the defective newborn.[24] Anger, frustration, and discomfort are alleged to make parents who have borne and may have to raise a severely impaired child emotionally unsuited for the critical medical decisions at hand.

Some commentators also raise a conflict of interest objection to lodging principal decision-making authority in the hands of parents of defective newborns.[25] The precise claim is that parents will be strongly influenced by factors other than the well-being of the infant—economic and emotional burdens on the parents, disruption of the family, and possible adverse impact on the parents' healthy children. Sources also point out that parents have not had the opportunity to develop the same kind of loving bond to a defective newborn that would be expected to be found with respect to infants and children generally.

These various arguments against parental responsibility have not altered the basic legal structure under which parents have initial authority to make medical decisions for their children, including life and death decisions for defective newborns. No court or legislature has altered or even seriously challenged the prevailing decision-making pattern. In fact, several of the most recent lower court expressions reaffirm parental authority to make critical determinations for defective newborns.[26] These decisions reflect a judicial willingness to leave initial decision-making "within privacy of the family relationship" so long as the decisions are made in consultation with medical sources. Even where legislative sources have sought to restrict the circumstances in which defective newborns may be allowed to die, no change is made in the allocation of authority to parents. The legislative effort has been to change the standards, but not the locus, of decision-making. (That effort will be discussed at the end of this chapter.)

Adherence to the principle of parental dominion does not mean that parents have unbridled discretion to withhold or withdraw life-preserving treatment from their defective infants. There is widespread awareness in medical and legal circles that dangers of ill-considered parental decisions do exist. But the principal response is not to remove parental responsibility, but rather to encourage review of decisions to ensure that substantive guidelines are followed and that abuse of parental authority is averted.

The presumptive starting point continues to be that parents can overcome the emotional trauma associated with the birth of a defective infant sufficiently to make an informed judgment about the infant's fate. It is recognized that medical personnel must provide careful consultation, and also that the parents should be afforded the maximum available time to ponder the decision. The underlying assumption also continues to be that parents by and large will act unselfishly, with concern for the infant the dominant factor in their decision-making. The rationale for reviewing parental decisions rather than displacing the parental decision-making role has been stated by the United States Supreme Court in another context (decisions to institutionalize disturbed children):

> [H]istorically, it has [been] recognized that natural bonds of affection lead parents to act in the best interests of their children. . . . [E]xperience and reality may rebut what the law accepts as a starting point; the incidence of child neglect and abuse cases attests to this. That some parents 'may at times be acting against the interests of their children' . . . creates a basis for caution, but is hardly a reason to discard wholesale those pages of human experience that teach that parents generally do act in the child's best interests. . . . The statist notion that governmental power should supersede parental authority in all cases because some parents abuse and neglect children is repugnant to American tradition.[27]

A central issue thus becomes not whether parents can be accorded authority to decline life-preserving treatment for a defective newborn, but what review mechanisms will be employed to scrutinize such decisions. The first stage of review is always the professional staff in the hospital's neonatal unit. That is, the surrounding health care professionals "bear responsibility to ensure that decision-making practices are adequate," to quote the recent President's Commission.[28] This effectively means that the staff must not simply acquiesce in seemingly aberrational parental decisions and must force further scrutiny of such decisions.

There is increasing sentiment that the next step in "further scrutiny" of a controversial parental determination should be through an intra-institutional review mechanism, probably some form of hospital ethics committee. Recommendations to this effect have come from the President's Commission, the American Academy of Pediatrics, at least one of the courts which have addressed the case of a defective newborn,[29] and several commentators. The federal government has 'also given impetus to the movement toward institutional infant care review committees. Both regulations adopted by the Department of Health and Human Services (HHS) in 1984 and legislation passed by Congress in the same year (amendments to the Child Abuse and Protection Act) call for HHS to encourage formation of internal hospital committees to cope with treatment issues surrounding defective newborns.[30]

The precise size, composition, and function of the ethics committee remains open for debate (as was the case with ethics committees dealing with incompetent adult patients). But there seems to be some concensus that the functions should include formulation of institutional policies toward defective infants' cases, education of hospital personnel, and review of controversial treatment decisions, all with a view toward discouraging and preventing decisions to terminate treatment which are thought to surpass prescribed bounds.[31]

There also appears to be some concensus that the ethics committee should be multi-disciplinary rather than strictly medical. A "model" committee, formulated by HHS based on suggestions by the American Academy of Pediatrics (AAP), calls for membership of at least seven persons, including a pediatric practitioner, a practicing nurse, a hospital administrator, a lawyer, a representative of a disability group, a lay community person, and a chairperson from the hospital medical staff. AAP guidelines dated August 1984 suggest, as well, participation by an expert in developmental disability and by a parent of a disabled child. At Jacobi Hospital in Bronx, N.Y., the review committee consists of doctors, a lawyer, an ethicist, a rehabilitation specialist, social workers, nurses, administrators, and community members. (That particular committee meets monthly to retrospectively review decisions involving defective newborns.) The multi-disciplinary composition of such committees reflects awareness that a decision regarding life-preserving treatment for a defective newborn may not be a purely medical matter.

One threshhold question regarding intra-institutional review is whether to require scrutiny of all determinations to withhold life-preserving treatment from a defective newborn. Reliance could be placed on the attending physician and professional staff as the natural advocates of the infant. The assumption would then be that the staff would turn to an institutional committee for guidance in any case that is really problematic. Yet, while medical personnel are generally oriented toward preservation of life, there are some indications that medical personnel may not be staunch enough patient advocates when left to their own devices. The medical literature reflects some instances where parental determinations were not contested despite apparent deviations from acceptable norms (e.g., the well-known "Johns Hopkins" case involving a mongoloid infant), as well as surprising antipathy on the part of some physicians toward any infant's potential existence which includes significant mental impairment. Surveys of pediatricians also indicate that physicians are extremely unlikely to rock the boat and seek judicial review of a parental decision with which they disagree. The reality is that many physicians empathize with the parental spectre of burden and isolation in raising a severely impaired child—sometimes to the point of too readily acquiescing in a nontreatment decision.

In light of all this, it might be advisable to require institutional scrutiny (at least post hoc review) of most decisions to allow defective infants to die. Both the model committee envisioned by the AAP task force and the model recommended by recent federal regulations view the institutional committee's principal role as offering educated counsel to families and physicians alike.[32] But according to the AAP task force, prospective review by the committee would be mandatory where withholding of life-sustaining care is proposed, unless the infant faces imminent death regardless. And while the HHS guidelines mention "internal review," without specifying whether the review must always be before the fact, the implication is that such review ought to be prior review if a decision to forego life-sustaining care is contemplated.[33] Those guidelines do hold out the possibility that certain classes of cases can eventually be defined in which committee review could be omitted.

In no instance does the recommended consultation, scrutiny, or review by an internal hospital committee purport to displant the decision-making authority of parents in conjunction with physicians. The hospital committee is not given veto authority; its approval is not a precondition to a treatment or nontreatment decision. Its presence would provide useful expert consultation, and its review would guarantee some exposure of critical decisions to neutral persons (those not immediately involved with or affected by the decision). The expectation is that if the committee discerns an inappropriate evaluation of an infant's interests, the committee will report to hospital officials. Hospital officials will then be expected to turn either to a court for judicial guidance, or to the state child protection agency.[34] Those favoring wide parental choice will resent scrutiny by a committee and potential interference with a parental preference. But an internal committee would seem to serve a useful scrutiny function, at least until more widespread understanding emerges as to the kinds of cases in which life-preserving care can appropriately be omitted.

A few commentators would go further and insist on judicial rather than institutional scrutiny of all decisions to withhold life-preserving treatment to a defective infant.[35] The argument is that only a court can provide the impartiality, consistency, and fairness needed in this setting of delicate life and death determinations. Yet, as was the case with dying adults, judicial resolution of every terminal decision would be neither feasible nor desirable. The judicial process, even when administered on an expedited basis, is simply too cumbersome, expensive, and time-consuming to be applied on a regular basis. In one recent case in which judicial machinery was invoked (because the infant had been abandoned and no parents were available), the court held hearings on five different occasions over four months and then advised that further proceedings could be held if the infant's condition should significantly change.[36] In the Baby Jane Doe case in New York, involving a challenge to a parental decision not to authorize surgery for a spina bifida infant, the highest state appellate court sadly lamented that the parents had been forced to undergo lengthy and expensive litigation.[37] At that point, the parents had been forced to litigate their treatment decision in three levels of state judicial tribunals over a period of several months. That was even before the federal Health and Human Services Administration initiated additional proceedings in federal court. That same case, with its massive and imprecise publicity, also illustrated how the glare of public proceedings can result in harassment and embarrassment to conscientious parents, as well as posing a significant burden to health professionals. In short, it would appear preferable to leave regularized review to internal hospital processes and to reserve judicial scrutiny for the individual cases in which the parental decision seems to be deviating from acceptable norms. We can now turn to an examination of those norms applicable to medical decisions involving defective newborns.

Standards for Decision-Making Affecting Defective Newborns

Interests of the Infant

As noted at the outset of this chapter, courts are beginning to acknowledge that there are exceptional circumstances in which life-sustaining medical treatment may be withheld from a defective newborn. Indeed, there are very few sources who would assert that there are *no* circumstances in which treatment may be withheld. Most commentators—even those extremely sensitive to life as a supreme value—concede there are situations in which the infant's prospects are so dismal that common sense and humanity demand relinquishing the life in question. The task then becomes defining the circumstances in which infants may be allowed to die. This means establishing a standard to guide the parents and physicians who, in conjunction, constitute the primary decision-makers.

In two recent decisions—one in Florida involving a permanently comatose infant and one in Massachusetts involving a child with congenital heart problems—the courts purported to apply a substituted judgment standard.[38] That is, they sought to decide what the infant would want done under the circumstances, if the infant were competent to decide. This appears to be a misguided approach. Prior discussion has emphasized that substituted judgment for incompetent patients is grounded on notions of individual autonomy and free choice. That doctrine seems inapplicable in the case of an infant who has not yet developed a value system or set of preferences which might guide assessment of personal wishes. [39] An infant has simply never had the competence on which autonomous decision-making is based. And defective infants, unlike moribund adults, have no prior life experience to serve as a yardstick for expectations and tolerable living conditions.

Putting aside the "substituted judgment" approach involving the patient's particularized preferences, the judicially developed standards for decision-making for a defective newborn are likely to be remarkably similar to those evolving in the context of incompetent adults. As in the case of the never competent adult, the primary guide is likely to be the best interests of the patient. That standard has commonly been employed in the context of a guardian making decisions on behalf of an incompetent ward. While the parent-child relationship is not a perfect analogue to the typical guardian-ward relation, there are increasing indications that the "best interests" standard is adaptable to life and death medical decisions involving defective newborns.

In the first place, a number of different courts (though not all) have employed the best interests notion in adjudicating petitions to overturn parental decisions rejecting medical treatment allegedly necessary for the life or well-being of a defective child.[40] That is, some courts have looked to the best interests of the child in determining the legal bounds of a parent's responsibility for the medical well-being of a child. In addition, important voices in the medical community have suggested that the best interests of the infant furnish the principal guide to medical decision-making in this context. For example, the Judicial Council of the American Medical Association has ruled:

> In the making of decisions for the treatment of seriously deformed
> newborns . . . the primary consideration should be what is best for the

individual patient. . . . Life should be cherished despite disabilities and handicaps, except when prolongation would be inhumane and unconscionable.[41]

Similarly, guidelines formulated by the Committee on Bioethics of the American Academy of Pediatrics stress that life-sustaining care can be withheld only where it serves the interests of the individual patient.[42] Finally, a number of commentators, most notably the recent President's Commission, have also endorsed "best interests of the infant" as the governing legal standard for decision-making.[43]

A child's best interests are usually equated with life. Many cases exist where neglect statutes or even homicide laws were applied to parents who failed to furnish medical assistance to infants.[44] Nonetheless, there appear to be some circumstances in which the infant's own interests dictate or permit a decision to withhold or withdraw life-sustaining medical intervention. Isolating those situations is not easy. Application of the best interests standard to defective newborns is inevitably a difficult task. Even with advanced diagnostic tools, medical predictions about the eventual degree of physical and mental impairment (to say nothing of survival itself) are imprecise. In most cases, decision-makers are forced to deal with probabilities rather than certainties or even near certainties. Furthermore, assessing either physical or psychic suffering for an infant can be a Herculean task. Pain is impossible to measure, particularly when emanating from a noncommunicative individual. Moreover, the feelings and experiences of infants are essentially unfathomable. "No one, especially normal, healthy adults, can 'place' themselves in a defective newborn's position and view life from that perspective."[45] And yet, the purported "burdens" on handicapped infants are inevitably assessed from the distorted perspective of healthy adults with considerable life experience. At the very least, these facts dictate some humility and caution on the part of persons deciding the fate of a defective newborn.

These admonitions notwithstanding, it is submitted that there are, in fact, circumstances when the discernible best interests of a defective infant warrant withholding of life-sustaining medical treatment. The first class of such cases is the "terminally ill" infant. As in the case of some adults facing a torturous and irremediable dying process, some severely incapacitated infants are born dying—with a prognosis that unavoidable death will occur within months or at most a year, and without any prospect of relief through medical intervention. In such instances, aggressive medical intervention may simply prolong a difficult dying process. Indeed, treatment may itself cause morbidity or iatrogenic consequences which exacerbate the already difficult dying process. In such instances, it is acknowledged by many sources that the best interests of the infant may well dictate withholding of vigorous medical treatment and the supplying instead of palliative or comforting care to ease the dying process.[46]

One disease category which fits the above profile is congenital heart disease so severe as to be untreatable. A Massachusetts court recently addressed the case of a four and one-half month old infant suffering from cyanotic heart disease (inadequate flow of oxygenated blood to the lungs) as well as lung blockage. The prognosis was death within a year. The court endorsed entry of a nonresuscitation or no code order, so that the child would not be revived after the first bout with coronary failure. Resuscitation would leave the dying infant in an even weaker and more feeble condition than his present one, and would carry a risk of causing additional pain as well as neurological and/or liver damage. The court found that resuscitation "would do nothing but prolong the child's agony and suffering" and would constitute a pointless or cruel "prolongation of the act of dying."[47]

Sometimes, an infant's terminal illness augers a protracted dying process entailing progressive neurological and physical deterioration. Tay-Sachs disease surfaces in infants at about age six months; from that point on it produces increasingly severe spasticity, dementia, and pain until an inevitable death by age five. Withholding of life-preserving medical measures, including artificial nutrition, may well be in a Tay-Sachs child's best interests at some stage in the deterioration process. Similarly, an infant whose gastrointestinal tract has been removed (after volvulus and infarction) can be preserved on a central venous catheter for a maximum of two years. The serious question in each instance is whether it is in the infant's interest to survive "tethered to an infusion pump" for that period, or whether an inevitable dying process is being needlessly prolonged.

Another class of cases—also parallel to incompetent adult cases—is that of the permanently comatose infant, the infant with no chance of ever reaching a cognitive state. Even if the comatose existence is preservable for a long period, no benefit is forthcoming to the vegetative patient and life-preserving treatment may be omitted or withdrawn. In other words, the principle of the *Quinlan* case is applicable to the realm of infants and children. This was the conclusion in a Florida case involving a ten month old infant who had been born asphyxiated and whose brain tissue had been ninety percent destroyed. The court upheld a parental decision to withdraw a respirator in light of the prognosis that the infant would never gain cognitive function.[48] A variety of causes can prompt infants or young children to suffer from PVS (persistent vegetative state).[49] Subject to medical verification of permanency coma, such infants may be relieved from their indefinite and irremediable limbo. On the same rationale, an infant suffering from anencephaly (absence of brain tissue) need not be given life-sustaining medical treatment. These infants have no possibility of cognitive awareness or interaction with their environment.

Some legal and medical commentators would go beyond the situation of the permanently comatose, totally noncognitive infant and impose a further "quality of life" parameter in the form of minimum mental capacity to enjoy a meaningful existence. This threshold is sometimes phrased as sufficient developmental potential for "social interaction" or "human relationships" or "capacity to love or be loved." One source has suggested that any infant can be allowed to expire if there is "no reasonable expectation that the infant will ever be able to respond affectively and cognitively to human attention and caring or engage in communication with others."[50]

There are serious problems with using limited intellectual function, by itself, as a determinative line for purposes of sustaining defective newborns. In the first place, the notion of "meaningful" capacity, or a life "worth living," is subject to arbitrary definition. One source would fix a thirty I.Q. as the guideline, others would admit that there is no objective criterion to measure capacity for human interaction. Moreover, even with devices such as CAT scans and EEG's, prediction of the eventual mental development of a newborn infant is a problematic task. (In a 1981 case, two physicians recommended withholding surgery on a spina bifida infant "likely" to be severely retarded. A court nonetheless ordered surgery and it turned out that the infant was not retarded.)[51] Most importantly, it is not clear that even the profoundly retarded child is excluded from all ability to interact with an environment, and thereby to secure some possible benefit from existence. We simply don't know what such a being is experiencing. And as long as best interests of the infant is the applicable standard, benefit to the infant must be assessed primarily from the infant's perspective. As in the case of incompetent adults, then, intellectual disfunction, by itself, ought not to be a basis for termination of treatment so long as the infant has some cognitive ability.

Other factors can and must be considered along with intellectual impairment in order to assess the best interests of a defective infant. Physical impairments, immobility, sensory deprivation, inability to maintain basic hygiene, and intrusive machinery or repeated medical procedures have all been cited as considerations. Thus, it is at least relevant that an infant will be not only severely retarded, but blind and deaf, partially paralysed, incontinent, and unable to leave a bed.

Yet in using these various factors to assess best interests of a defective infant, it must be remembered that the overall standard is not "potential for a reasonably happy and productive life" as some sources would suggest, but rather net interests of the human being. This means that allowing a defective infant to die can only be justified where "the negative experiences—the physical pain and psychological suffering that would occur in continued living—would outweigh the positive experiences and pleasures that would occur."[52] Stated differently, the impairments of an infant must be so severe that death is preferable to continued existence.[53]

This is essentially the same standard of net burdens and benefits described in *Conroy* as applicable to incompetent, dying adults. The problem lies in applying the standard to the defective newborn. For the standard presupposes that parents and physicians can somehow balance the benefits and burdens of the prospective handicapped existence despite uncertainties in prognosis and difficulties in assessing the feelings and experiences of these noncommunicative beings. Some authorities question this initial premise. They contend that an infant's degree of discomfort or concomitant benefit within a diminished quality of life is basically unmeasurable. Their conclusion is that medical intervention ought to be mandatory so long as any significant period of existence can be preserved, regardless of the supposed suffering accompanying that existence.[54]

Certainly, there is need in assessing the best interests of defective newborns to avoid what Professor Robert Weir has labelled "adult elitism."[55] This is a tendency to attribute adult perceptions of harm or detriment to infants who have never had the experiences or expectations of adults. In other words, infants who have never known certain qualities of life may not suffer from their absence in the way that some adults assume. An infant (or child) may not be disappointed with sensory deprivation if he has no learned expectations. An infant may not suffer from loneliness in the acute way of someone who has previously enjoyed human company. And an infant may not suffer the frustrations of immobility or the embarrassments of incontinence in the way that a person accustomed to a normal lifestyle would.[56] In short, adult decision-makers must take care not to ascribe to an infant perceptions, emotions, and suffering characteristic of a mature adult who has never experienced physical disability.

Given the uncertainties of prognosis and the difficulties of assessing either negative or positive feelings of an infant, the hypothesis must be that continued living is in the best interests of the vast majority of defective newborns. Nonetheless, there are cases in which decision-makers can reasonably conclude that the infant's prospective existence is so distressing and miserable that the withholding of life-sustaining treatment is indeed in the infant's best interests. Some infants afflicted with congenital heart problems or chronic pulmonary disease, for example, may be fated to such constant respiratory distress and dependence on a variety of machines as to make severance from the machines a form of permanent relief. Similarly, a victim of Lesch-Nyhan disease, marked by severe retardation and compulsive self-mutilation, may offer an example where life preservation is not in the infant's own best interests. I will not attempt to catalogue the disease categories in which an afflicted infant's best interests may well be served by withholding life-preserving treatment. Each infant's status and prospects must ultimately be assessed on a case by case basis, with particular focus on physical and emotional suffering inevitably facing the patient. Though there are no mechanical ways to measure pain, medical personnel and parents may be able to instinctively sense that some infants are experiencing intractable pain. Moreover, it is a fair assumption that infants must suffer from being prodded, plied, and subjected to intrusive and repetitive medical interventions. Thus, there will be some instances when a defective newborn's condition presages such unrelievable suffering that any possible positive experiences are outweighed. In such instances, the normal presumption in favor of preserving life is overcome.

An interesting variation on the theme of "best interests" occurs when parents of handicapped infants or children opt for "conservative medical treatment"—choosing limited medical intervention through which the infant's life is saved, but the potential life span of the infant is significantly abridged (compared to the maximum life span obtainable through aggressive medical intervention). The conservative course of treatment is rationalized by saying that aggressive treatment (usually surgery) would carry some mortal risk (i.e., a chance that the infant might not survive the surgery), or would risk causing some negative complications or aggravations to the quality of life of the defective newborn. To complete the argument, it is asserted that parents have the prerogative of selecting among recommended medical options.[57]

An example of this conservative approach was the Baby Jane Doe case litigated in New York in 1983 and 1984. Baby Jane Doe was born on October 11, 1983, suffering from multiple birth defects including hydrocephalus, microcephaly (abnormally small head), and spina bifida, with accompanying impaired bladder, rectal, leg and sensory functioning. The prognosis was that she would be severely retarded, epileptic, paralyzed, bedridden, incontinent, and unable to communicate with persons around her.[58] With surgery to close the lesion on her back (to avoid infection) and to install a shunt to drain excess fluids from the skull, Baby Jane Doe's projected life span was twenty years. This was one medical option.

Another medical opinion favored antibiotic treatment (but not surgery) to prevent infection. With the latter course of treatment, the projected life span was a maximum of two years. (Without any medical intervention, the infant would probably have died within a couple of months.) The recommendation against surgery was apparently based in part on a risk that surgery would remove whatever slight movement of the lower extremities was possible; resultant total paralysis would then necessitate certain intubations which would risk causing infections in the urinary tract and bladder.

Baby Jane Doe's parents chose "conservative" treatment—nutrition, antibiotics, and dressing of the exposed spinal sac—rather than surgery. A hospital employee was apparently disturbed by the parental choice and notified persons outside the hospital. A petition was then filed seeking a court order for surgery. The petitioner, a lawyer and right to life advocate, claimed that the parental failure to arrange surgery constituted child neglect. On October 19, eight days after the birth, a trial court judge ordered surgery. The parents appealed and on October 21, the state Appellate Division reversed.[59] Noting that the medical treatment chosen posed no imminent danger of death to the infant, the appellate court ruled that the parents had simply "chosen one course of appropriate medical treatment over another."[60] The conservative course was "well within accepted medical standards" so that the parent's decision could reasonably be deemed to be in the best interests of the infant.

The parents continued to visit and hold Baby Jane Doe. An attack of meningitis was overcome by antibiotics. By April 1984, the spinal lesion had apparently closed by itself and an operation to install a shunt had been authorized by the parents and performed in order to make the infant "more comfortable." The parents then took Baby Jane Doe home.[61] In the meantime, efforts by right to life supporters to secure intervention from New York's Child Protection Services and from the federal Department of Health and Human Services had failed.[62]

The Baby Jane Doe case was probably rightly decided, in terms of result, but perhaps for the wrong reasons. In the first place, the fact that the conservative treatment avoided placing the infant in an immediately life-threatening position should not be determinative. While Professor Joseph Goldstein of Yale has argued strenuously that government intervention in parental medical decision-making ought to be impermissible in the absence of an imminent threat to a child's life,[63] that view has not prevailed. Judicial intervention on the basis of child neglect can generally be grounded on any medical decision which threatens "serious harm" to a child.[64] And a significant diminution in a child's projected life span is certainly serious harm.

Courts are, in fact, reluctant to find child neglect where a parental choice of treatment does not provoke an immediately life-threatening situation.[65] But this policy is in part based on considerations not present in Baby Jane Doe's case. Sometimes, a court will assume that the parents have merely chosen interim treatment, and that more aggressive treatment will be forthcoming if the child patient's condition worsens.[66] Sometimes, a court will withhold intervention on the basis that the child will soon reach sufficient maturity to make an independent decision about non life-threatening problems. Neither of these situations was present in Baby Jane Doe's case. As noted, the reality is that courts will, in fact, intervene even with regard to situations that are not life-threatening medical conditions if the parental choice of treatment threatens serious harm and is so arbitrary as to show disregard for a child's best interests.[67]

Nor should it be determinative in a case like Baby Jane Doe's that there was some risk of morbidity (increased paralysis and infection) accompanying the surgical intervention, or that there was some responsible medical opinion favoring the conservative course of treatment. These facts are highly relevant to the scrutiny of the parental choice of treatment, but they are not by themselves determinative of whether child neglect exists. True, parents must inevitably weigh possible side effects and possible fatal risks while considering a course of medical treatment for a child. Those risks might be so substantial as to justify a determination to forego a particular medical procedure. Thus, parents have on occasion been upheld in decisions to omit corrective surgery for crippling conditions in children where the surgery posed some fatal risk to the child.[68] Similarly, it is normally a parental prerogative to assess the soundness of conflicting medical opinions on diverse treatments. This deference is accorded to parental judgment both out of respect for traditional family structure, and because no government agency can, as a practical matter, substitute its judgment for that of parents. Not only are the potential cases too numerous, but the imponderables being weighed—variations in quality of existence versus risks of morbidity or death—are not suited for simple second guessing of parental decisions.[69]

These caveats about parental prerogatives notwithstanding, a parental choice of medical treatment is reviewable pursuant to child neglect statutes and is overrideable where the decision is so unreasonable as to be arbitrary. Thus, while a shunt for a hydrocephalic infant might carry some risk of infection and even death, the benefits—relief of pressure on the brain and avoidance of further retardation—are so great that a court would in most cases override a parental rejection of the surgical procedure.[70] Moreover, the presence of some medical support for a treatment does not preclude judicial intervention to order an alternative treatment carrying much wider medical support and much better chances of aiding a stricken child.[71] This is true even if the treatment ordered by the court would entail some side effects avoidable through the course of treatment chosen by the parents. A "correct" medical decision is largely a matter of probabilities and degrees—chances of a cure or remission through each of the proposed treatments, extent of potential benefit, probability of a particular risk materializing, and severity of the feared adverse side effects in each instance.[72] Where a parental decision is reasonable it will be upheld. But where parents' overall assessment seems arbitrary, the parental choice is subject to being overturned as being inconsistent with the best interests of the child.

Applying these lessons to the Baby Jane Doe case, the presence of some medical advice to rely on antibiotic treatment does not, by itself, establish that such a course was reasonably in the best interests of the infant. More data would ordinarily have to be provided about the degree and significance of the risks involved in surgery. Normally, a gain of many years of potential existence would outweigh a risk of a minor increase in an already virtually complete paralysis, or a risk of infection controllable with routine medical means. If Baby Jane Doe had the potential for normal intellectual development (as some spina bifida babies do), it is implausible that a court would accept in a neglect proceeding a parental medical decision which, for the sake of avoiding manageable side effects such as infection, reduces an infant's life span by ten or fifteen years. A responsible physician's recommendation supporting the parental decision is relevant evidence supporting the reasonableness of that decision, but it is not determinative. A court can conceivably decide that a medical recommendation (and parental decision) are not consistent with an infant's best interests and appoint a temporary guardian to make the critical medical decision. In short, conservative medical treatment may or may not be in the best interests of a defective infant, depending on the circumstances of each case.

Perhaps implicit in the New York court's upholding of the parents' decision to reject life-extending surgery was a judgment that the quality of Baby Jane Doe's life was so dismal that any treatment which merely extended life without improving the patient's condition could not be in her best interests. Indeed, one judicial opinion connected with the case reported that there was an extremely high risk that she would be "so severely retarded that she could never interact with her environment or with other people."[73] A commentator on the case has claimed that Baby Jane Doe was so disabled that she would be "conscious of little except pain."[74] These reports trigger the question whether even antibiotic treatment should have been administered. The parents, in the harsh glare of publicity and a pending court case, chose a path labelled "conservative treatment." This included administration of antibiotics to combat meningitis and later installation of a shunt to relieve pressure from hydrocephalus. But if it was really in Baby Jane Doe's best interests to withhold surgery and to shorten her life prospects so appreciably, one must wonder whether it was in her best interests to undertake life-preserving treatment of any form.

The Interests of Others—Parents, Siblings, and Society

Ordinarily, parents are responsible for the care and nurture of their offspring. This legal and moral responsibility is imposed even though child rearing may involve significant emotional and financial impositions on the parents. The rationale is simple. The parents chose to bring a helpless and innocent life into being. They can reap the pleasures of child rearing, but they must also assume the burdens.

The raising of a severely handicapped child, however, normally poses extraordinary emotional, physical, and financial burdens on the parents and siblings of the child. Tending to the needs of a severely handicapped child can take a considerable toll on the time and energies of those responsible. One cost may be increased tension and internal conflict among family members. This emotional toll may be reflected in an increased incidence of divorce, or in behavioral problems among siblings of the handicapped child.

The economic toll accompanying multidisciplinary care for the child can also be considerable. Families may fear lifelong economic bondage. Their frustration may be increased by the realization that these potential burdens could have been entirely averted if, a scant four months before the fateful birth, they had realized the fetus' condition and obtained an abortion.

The central question becomes whether the extraordinary potential burdens upon a family can legitimately be considered by decision-makers in deciding the fate of a severely defective newborn. Up to this point, I have assumed that the governing standard for decision-making is the best interests of the infant, and that those interests don't include the possible burdens upon surrounding family members.

That assumption at least deserves examination. For it is very clear that in the real world decision-makers are sometimes influenced by the potential impact on the family of a severely defective newborn. For example, in two widely reported instances in which parents opted to forego surgery to remove feeding blockages from mongoloid infants—the "Johns Hopkins" case in Maryland and the "Infant Doe" case in Indiana—concern for the siblings of the defective newborns apparently played a significant role in the decisions.[75] Other anecdotal reports confirm that some parents declining treatment for spina bifida infants are influenced by the prospective long-term stress upon the family unit.[76] Further, the 1976 survey of pediatricians cited above revealed that fifty-six percent of the surgeons and forty-one percent of the pediatric physicians viewed the family's interests as a first priority factor in making critical decisions for defective newborns.[77] Some physicians feel that even if a family could manage to adjust to the stress of a severely defective child, the family's resources would be better utilized if devoted to the healthy children.[78]

A number of commentators—medical, legal, and philosophical—claim that the impact on the family constitutes an important and legitimate factor for consideration in shaping the defective newborn's treatment.[79] Their point is that parents and siblings have interests that are as substantial and deserving of consideration as those of the defective infant. Their conclusion is usually that family interests may be allowed to prevail when a "heavy burden" would fall on the family from survival of a severely impaired infant. One formulation would require, for the family interest to prevail, "such unusual expense and emotional involvement on the part of parents that the continued existence of the family unit is itself placed in serious jeopardy."[80]

From a moral perspective, the legitimacy of family interests is readily understandable. Through no fault of their own, the parents appear to be facing an enduring hardship. Fate seems to have dealt these parents a bad hand. And, if they had known only a few months before that the infant would be born severely impaired, they could have aborted the fetus and avoided all the turmoil now facing them. Nonetheless, the consequence of a nontreatment decision based on avoiding burdens to the family may be the death of a defective newborn. Can avoidance of burdens to parents and siblings serve as a legal justification for ending that newborn's life? The answer appears to be "no" under most circumstances.

The right of parents to protect family emotional and economic interests does not ordinarily encompass termination of a human life. Of course, there are some philosophical observers who contend that a newborn infant does not enjoy full human and moral status.[81] These sources claim that full moral status is achieved by an infant only with self-awareness or a concept of self, a point supposedly reached only weeks after birth. If a newborn were indeed not entitled to personhood, it might then follow that "the parents' life plans should not be ruined or the quality of their lives seriously impaired just to keep alive an infant who is (at best) a potential person."[82] A newborn might be treated, in effect, like a fetus subject to abortion.

Whatever the moral appeal of this position, and I by no means endorse it, it has no basis in law. That is, an infant in every American jurisdiction is entitled to full personhood from the moment of birth. In the famous abortion decisions of 1973, the Supreme Court ruled that a state's interest in potential life could not override a woman's interest in deciding whether to bear a child until the fetus was viable (at about the twenty-fourth week of pregnancy). From the point of viability onward, a state could choose to protect the fetus. If a viable fetus can be protected against destruction, it is certain that a newborn can be similarly protected. The Supreme Court purported not to decide whether life begins at conception, or at viability, referring instead to fetal existence as potential life. But there is no question that the Court regarded live birth as a mark of personhood. In fact, every newborn is treated by American criminal, constitutional, tort, and family law as entitled to the status of a person.[83]

The fact that a newborn is a person does not automatically fix the extent of affirmative obligation owed to it by parents or any other source. The extent to which parents must undertake extensive burdens in order to preserve a defective newborn is determined by the law of child neglect and homicide. (The possible contention that the federal constitutional concept of "familial privacy" affects parental responsibility toward defective newborns will be examined later.)

As previously noted, child neglect laws generally impose upon parents—the persons who brought an innocent and helpless life into being—a legal obligation to provide life-sustaining medical care. This obligation applies, at least, until the parents have arranged suitable alternative custody for the child. (And even if a parent can turn over custody to an appropriate state agency, some financial responsibility usually remains until the child is legally adopted.) There is no indication either in statute or case law that the parental obligation is qualified according to the I.Q. or impaired abilities of an infant. Nor does emotional or financial burdensomeness of a child normally provide an exemption from parental obligations. There is no question, for example, that parents are legally responsible for a child who is obstreperous and incorrigible, despite the emotional and economic stress placed on the parents. Likewise, parental obligations toward a "normal" child would not change just because the child became severely disabled as a result of an accident or other trauma.

The sole justification for withholding life-sustaining treatment which emerges from the cases on child neglect is when it is in the "best interests of the child." In speaking to those best interests, the cases relating to defective infants appear to focus on the personal interests of the child and don't refer to the burdens posed upon parents and siblings.[84] By implication from this silence, judicial precedent seems to exclude family interests from the category of best interests of the child/patient. Most commentators, including the President's Commission, support this interpretation of judicial authority. These sources regard the "best interests of the child" standard as excluding consideration of a defective infant's potential impact upon parents and siblings.[85] The Judicial Council of the American Medical Association has urged that the deformed newborn's best interests deserve primary consideration. The implication seems to be that the potential burdens upon family or society are to receive little, if any, attention in treatment decisions.[86] A similar position was adopted by the American Academy of Pediatricians (AAP). That body stressed that a defective infant's interests form the "primary obligation" in decision-making, and that withdrawal of life-preserving care can't be prompted by concern for the well-being of surrounding family members.[87]

There is some oblique support for the proposition that extraordinary fiscal burdens on parents flowing from medical treatment of a defective newborn might justify a decision to withhold life-preserving care. Though the precedents on defective infants don't generally refer to the issue, some limit to fiscal burdens upon parents is probably part of the calculus of defining child neglect. That is, it is probably understood that parents need not pauperize themselves in order to provide medical treatment for children. This notion is occasionally expressed explicitly in a child neglect statute. For example, the New York Family Court Act allows a finding of child neglect upon failure to provide surgical treatment only if the parent was "financially able to do so [provide treatment] or [was] offered financial or other reasonable means to do so."[88] Even where this financial exemption is not specifically included by statute, it is a concept probably implicit in the law of child neglect.

This principle permitting parents to avert crushing fiscal burdens in providing medical care should have limited impact on most life and death decisions regarding defective newborns. Often, the surgical procedures involved are relatively simple. Medicaid is available to cover the expenses for indigent persons. In other cases, hospitals appear to be willing to provide life-preserving treatment for infants, and to absorb the losses if the parents prove unable to pay.[89] Where the life-threatening condition can only be combatted through protracted and crushingly expensive treatment, and outside sources (hospital, government benefit programs, etc.) have not offerred to ease the burden, the implied fiscal limit on parental obligation might come into play. But the mere fact that after an affordable life-preserving medical procedure, the continued maintenance of the handicapped infant will impose economic burdens on the family is probably not enough to invoke the fiscal burden defense to child neglect. In short, the fiscal burden justification for omitting life-preserving treatment is applicable only where the immediate intervention poses insuperable financial problems for a family. This principle is as applicable to a "normal" child needing medical care as to a defective infant.

Professor Joseph Goldstein has advanced a more radical position. He asserts that society cannot force parents to preserve defective infants whose lives the parents consider not worth living unless government provides "the special financial, physical, and psychological resources" necessary to proper treatment of a handicapped child.[90] Thus, Professor Goldstein contends that the state must assume full fiscal responsibility for the special needs of any defective newborns whom parents are compelled to nurture against their better judgment.

Parents certainly have a moral claim that the extraordinary burdens of raising a severely handicapped child should be shared by society. But there is no corresponding legal claim against the state for fiscal resources—certainly no claim which can be enforced by sacrifice of the child's life. As Professor Robert Weir has observed: "in wishing that life were more fair, that burdens were more evenly distributed, . . . it is not justifiable to override a potential person's claim to life merely to save other persons trouble."[91] The parental obligation to preserve a handicapped infant's life cannot hinge on state assumption of burdens any more than preservation of a disabled adult dependent (such as a spouse severely injured in an auto accident, or a prematurely senile spouse) is contingent on government absorption of the costs, or on free provision of rehabilitative services. There is no constitutional principle which says that the government must either fund the burdens which it imposes on guardians responsible for maintaining dependents or must consent to the termination of the dependent's existence. Even if a third trimester (viable) fetus threatens to impose psychological and economic strain on a family, a mother is not constitutionally entitled to abort that fetus.[92]

All this is not to say that states ought not to provide much better assistance in the raising of handicapped children. The moral claim is strong for improved services for the education and care of handicapped persons. The point is simply that parents cannot legally justify withholding life-preserving treatment—other than according to the "best interests of the infant" standard—simply because the government has not fully provided for the special needs of handicapped children. Economic or health interests of parents or siblings can only be given significant weight in the rare instances when the infant's preservation will immediately and seriously jeopardize the health or economic survival of a family.

The argument for considering the potential burdens on parents and siblings is further weakened by the opportunity of parents to relinquish child-rearing responsibility by means short of withholding treatment to a defective newborn. In most jurisdictions, parents can opt to surrender custody and place a child up for adoption.[93] Because severely impaired children are hard to place, the surrendered child may end up in foster care or in a state institutional setting. Nonetheless, in all these instances the potential burdens on the parents of a severely defective infant are significantly alleviated. In light of the infant's normal strong interest in continued life, the parents' reduced potential burdens (where parents are free to renounce custody) can't justify parental withholding of life-preserving treatment.[94]

Many states would insist that even after surrendering the infant the parents must contribute toward the costs of institutional care. But these payments could be adjusted according to the financial ability of the parents. That way there would be no possibility of the kind of crushing economic burden which might justify withholding treatment.

Some parents might be reluctant to consign their offspring to a state institution for the handicapped. Some of these facilities are notorious for their inadequate attention to the needs of the handicapped residents. Professor Goldstein has branded the typical institutional setting available as "little more than storage space," and Dr. Raymond Duff refers to such institutions as "dying bins."[95]

The prospective conditions facing a defective newborn—whether in a foster care or institutional setting—are unquestionably relevant to the decision whether or not to forego life-preserving medical treament. For the prospective environment and extent of care available to a handicapped child are among the elements shaping the child's best interests. Thus, for a parent deciding a defective newborn's fate, the conditions of institutional care (if the child will likely be institutionalized) ought properly to be factored into the best interests calculus. The ultimate determination, however, is whether after weighing the net potential benefits and burdens facing the defective newborn, the infant patient's best interests would be served by withholding life-preserving care. In other words, the institutional environment must be so inadequate that, in light of the infant's impairments, the infant would be better off dead than warehoused in the institution.

I have argued in this section that, from a perspective of current legal doctrines, the emotional and financial impacts on a defective infant's family are not proper decision-making factors in most treatment situations. The applicable standard revolves around the best interests of the defective newborn. So long as the medical procedure needed does not pose a crushing financial burden, the economic toll on the family should not provide a defense to a child neglect petition. Nor does the prospective emotional burden on parents and siblings provide a justification for nontreatment of the newborn. The infant's interest in life normally prevails against the psychological toll on the family. Moreover, the parents can avoid most of the burdens in question by relinquishing legal custody of the child.

To some extent, these conclusions sound like "the moralistic conclusion[s] of the abstract theorist."[96] The prospective burdens on a family may be very real and very anguishing. (Surrender of custody may not be realistic because the parents would ultimately opt to provide a home environment, with all its burdens, rather than consigning the infant to a state institution.) The gains or benefits to a severely defective child may be hard to fathom, even if physical pain will not constantly plague its existence. A profoundly retarded individual cannot enjoy many of the satisfactions available to "normal" persons. Under those circumstances, physicians and judges understandably feel a moral ambivalence. The tangible interests of parents and siblings are jeopardized while the marginal existence preserved may not seem worth the sacrifice. Moral ambivalence is probably what prompts the instances in which physicians acquiesce in parental decisions to allow defective infants to die without careful application of a "best interests of the infant" standard. It does not surprise me that physicians' attitudes, and probably ongoing practices in hospitals as well, diverge from the legal model. I have no trouble concluding that "best interests of the infant" offers the only proper standard under current judicially evolved doctrine, and that pursuant to that standard the vast majority of defective newborns should be treated vigorously. Nonetheless, I personally have a lot of trouble envisioning myself signing an order which compels treatment for a severely defective infant against the wishes of parents.

Another factor which contributes to moral ambivalence in the salvaging of seriously defective infants is allocation of societal resources. The economic costs of neonatal intensive care are considerable. A study of

1,185 admissions to a neonatal intensive care unit between 1976 and 1978 disclosed an average cost of $8,069 per stay. In five instances, the costs exceeded $100,000 and in nineteen cases the costs fell between $50,000 and $100,000. For infants weighing between 500 and 1000 grams, the average cost was $28,128 and the daily charge was $1165.[97] (All these figures exclude the seven years of inflation since 1978.) It is not terribly unusual for charges associated with low birth weight infants to exceed $100,000.[98] In some instances, the infant expires despite vigorous medical efforts. If the infant survives but suffers from serious permanent handicaps, the postnatal costs of medical care and special education must be considered. A lifetime of institutional care, for example, totals many hundreds of thousands of dollars.

Only a small percentage of neonatal intensive care charges are borne by the parents out of pocket. The bulk is absorbed by private insurance, government benefit programs (i.e., taxpayers), and hospitals.[99] Many sources argue that the compulsion to preserve newborn life must be tempered by a duty to use limited resources soundly. The following quotations are typical:

> [I]f we do not look at the costs, which are high, and if we do not consider the best allocation of our limited resources, we are being irresponsible. There are no guidelines, much less a consensus, on whether it is appropriate to consider the financial cost of saving the life of a seriously ill, defective newborn.[100]

> One may admire families that devote their entire energies to the care of a severely handicapped family member, but it would hardly make sense for a society to act likewise. Some people's legitimate needs must be preferred over other people's equally legitimate needs.[101]

The conclusion among such commentators is usually that undue expense, or very costly procedures in return for small gain, must be averted.

On its face, the applicable "best interests of the infant" standard leaves no place for societal economic costs to come into play in individual treatment decisions. This is generally as it should be, for any social utilitarian calculus—measuring the resources to be expended against the worth of a life—would seem to jeopardize many impaired and helpless human beings. The plaint that communal resources could be better expended elsewhere is not ordinarily heeded in individual life or death decisions. Cost benefit analysis is reserved to less poignant situations.

The best interests standard to the contrary notwithstanding, awareness of economic burdens will almost inevitably influence medical decisions affecting defective newborns. For example, sound allocation of resources dictates a policy that very expensive medical intervention be withheld from an infant who cannot be salvaged for more than a few months. Even commentators who oppose virtually all selective treatment policies are willing to concede that vigorous treatment can be withheld if the infant can't be preserved for "an appreciable amount of time"— usually defined arbitrarily as about six months.[102] Implicit in that policy is an economic efficiency judgment that substantial resources should not be expended for so little gain. Similarly, most people are willing to base aggressive treatment decisions on *probabilities* of certain outcomes—an approach based in part on economic concerns. To cite an example, if there is a strong probability that a particular spina bifida infant will be profoundly retarded, many physicians will recommend against surgical intervention even though there is some chance that the infant's mental development will be much better than projected. In such instances, the knowledge that considerable resources would be expended with little chance of a successful outcome probably influences a decision to withhold surgery.

As in the case of incompetent adults, public funding sources will eventually refuse to fund medical interventions which pose no benefit to defective infants even if the parents or guardians would prefer to continue treatment. As classes of cases are identified in which vigorous treatment is deemed inconsistent with the best interests of a defective newborn, those cases will be excluded from public benefit programs. Candidates for exclusion include anencephaly, permanent coma, and spina bifida accompanied by certain complicating factors (gross hydrocephalus, total paralysis, etc.). The consequence will not be to require termination of treatment, but rather to withhold public financing of the nonbeneficial treatment.

The Role of Family Privacy and Parental Autonomy

In recent cases upholding parental decisions to terminate life-preserving treatment for defective newborns, the courts have referred to federal constitutional notions of family privacy and autonomy as supporting judicial nonintervention.[103] Yet in the prior section, the conclusion emerged that family interests are generally excluded from the determinative criterion of "best interests of the infant." It is important then to establish the precise relevance and impact of parents' constitutional interests on medical decision-making for defective newborns.

The United States Supreme Court has declared that natural parents have a fundamental liberty interest, pursuant to the Fifth and Fourteenth Amendments to the Constitution, "in the care, custody, and management of their children."[104] This liberty interest has been found to embody broad parental authority over a variety of decisions affecting minor children. Among the recognized areas of parental control are education, discipline, choice of medical therapy, and choice of institutional setting in which therapeutic care is to be administered.[105]

A variety of factors underlie this traditional respect for parental decision-making. Broad parental authority is thought to promote the family unit, which in turn is thought to cultivate a bonding and an intimacy conducive to child rearing. Given the diversity of values represented in family units, family decision-making autonomy also promotes a pluralistic, multi-cultural society. In addition, society allocates decisions to parents on the premise that "natural bonds of affection" lead parents generally to act to advance the welfare of their children. This is consistent with government's concern with protecting incompetent, helpless populations such as children. Finally, private familial decision-making is efficient. It's simply not practical for an outside source to supervise or second guess the plethora of decisions about clothing, shelter, education, entertainment, and health care which affect children in a family setting.

The rationale for respecting parental decision-making does not apply with full force to life and death decisions on behalf of defective newborns. The intimate bonds which are assumed to characterize family relations may not have matured toward an infant whose brief existence has been spent in a neonatal intensive care unit. The normal holding and fondling of the infant may well be precluded. Furthermore, the parents of the newborn have not yet undertaken the responsibilities and duties of child rearing which are normally a counterpart to the exercise of parental rights.[106] If parents opt to forego treatment and the infant will soon die, the customary link between parental duty and parental right is somewhat attenuated. But even if we assume that the constitutional interest in parental decision-making fully attaches from birth of a child, we must still factor in various limitations traditionally applied to parental rights to make decisions for their children.

Basic constitutional doctrine holds that the fundamental liberty interest in parental decision-making is by no means absolute. While parents are allowed to order family priorities and impose value preferences in a multitude of situations, there are limits to the autonomy accorded. Child labor laws, compulsory education, and vaccination requirements all constitute inroads on parental autonomy or family privacy.

Perhaps the most traditional limitation on parental decision-making is invoked whenever the health or safety of a child is significantly jeopardized. That is, the multitude of instances when parental choices prevail (even if detrimental to a child's interests) do not usually include life and death determinations. Anglo-American legal tradition has always accorded government a prerogative to act as guardian of legally incompetent and helpless persons whose health or safety is seriously threatened. This parens patriae notion is applied even against parents, at least in circumstances typically posing special hazards for the interests of children. For example, placement of a child in a mental hospital carries such risks of permanent stigma and harm that parental discretion has been circumscribed by a requirement of neutral medical review. The Supreme Court did not impose automatic judicial review on such hospitalization decisions, but the Court did mandate an independent medical determination that the child is emotionally ill and can benefit from the treatment being offered.[107] Another example of parens patriae intervention in parental decision-making involves sterilization of a minor. The obvious harm to children's potential procreation interests dictates careful scrutiny of any parental determination in favor of sterilization.[108] Sterilization will be allowed only if deemed to be in the best interests of the affected child.

In the context of medical decisions on behalf of defective newborns, the child neglect laws circumscribe the discretion of parents. Numerous cases have held that a parental failure to provide needed medical care, even if motivated by conscientious religious scruples, furnishes a basis for state intervention.[109] This intervention will be forthcoming whether the parental medical decision poses a mortal risk, or merely threatens serious injury to a child's well-being.[110] Certainly, the interest in parental privacy asserted in the context of impaired infants is not any constitutionally stronger than the interest in religious freedom which has failed in constitutional confrontations with a state interest in preserving a child's well-being in the face of a life-endangering threat.

There is no principle which diminishes the state's protective interest because the infant is impaired in some respect. This fact emerges clearly from cases which have overridden parental refusals to provide surgery for spina bifida infants.[111] The only situations in which parents have been allowed to forego critical treatment for infants is where the best interests of the infant were arguably served by the parental decision. In short, the constitutional concepts of parental autonomy and family privacy don't afford parents a broad substantive discretion to withhold life-preserving treatment for defective newborns.[112] Parents' medical choices are always limited by the best interests standard.

The only deference to parental discretion in the context of critical medical decisions for defective newborns comes in the scope of judicial or administrative review of a decision purporting to be in the best interests of the defective newborn. The intangible variables involved in every such decision—including medical estimates of mortality and morbidity risks, and assessments of the likely benefits and burdens of the prospective existence (with and without treatment)—suggest that parental decisions should not regularly be second-guessed. So long as a parental determination constitutes a good faith effort to further the best interests of the infant, and so long as the determination cannot be branded as arbitrary, parental judgment ought to be sustained.[113] Thus, parental nontreatment decisions (in cooperation with medical personnel) ought to prevail so long as it's plausible under the particular circumstances that the defective newborn will be better off without aggressive medical intervention. This deferential approach is consistent with past judicial willingness to reject neglect petitions grounded on nontreatment decisions where there was at least some plausible basis for the parental decision.[114]

Legislative Influences

The Federal Role

Up until 1982, the law relating to life-preserving treatment for defective newborns was thought to be shaped entirely by state and local legislative measures. Local homicide and/or child neglect statutes ostensibly determined the scope of parental responsibility toward newborn infants. The thrust of judicial decision-making pursuant to such legislative measures was described in the previous section.

In 1982, a powerful new element entered the picture. President Reagan asserted at that point that *federal* law (a statute barring discrimination against handicapped persons by institutions receiving federal funds) applies to decisions to withhold medical treatment from defective newborns, and that such federal law forbids the withholding of life-preserving treatment in most circumstances.

The immediate stimulus to this federal involvement was the Infant Doe case in Indiana in April 1982. In that instance, the Indiana courts refused to override a parental decision not to provide surgery to a Down's syndrome infant born with a correctible esophagal atresia. The infant was permitted to die from starvation. The case drew wide publicity and caught the attention of the White House. Within fifteen days of Infant Doe's death, President Reagan directed the Secretary of the Department of Health and Human Services (HHS) to notify federally funded health care providers that Section 504 of the Rehabilitation Act of 1973[115] forbids withholding medical services from handicapped infants that would be provided to nonhandicapped infants.[116]

The President relied on statutory language which broadly prohibited service programs receiving federal funds from discriminating "solely by reason of . . . handicap" against an "otherwise qualified handicapped individual. . . ." Mr. Reagan's contention was that a defective newborn was "handicapped" and that withholding of critical treatment was a form of prohibited "discrimination."

The Rehabilitation Act of 1973 was broadly aimed at providing rehabilitation and independent living to handicapped individuals by guaranteeing nondiscriminatory access to education, employment, and transportation facilities. There was no indication in the legislative history that Congress contemplated application of the Act to individual medical decisions. Early HEW regulations interpreting the Act had spoken about health care facilities, but apparently only with regard to providing handicapped persons unfettered access to the institutions.[117]

Despite this somewhat murky legislative background, HHS responded with alacrity to President Reagan's instructions. On May 18, 1982, HHS notified federally funded health care providers (a class including approximately 7,000 American hospitals) that Section 504 prohibited the withholding of treatment or nutrition from a handicapped infant unless such treatment was "medically contraindicated."[118] HHS followed this notice up with detailed regulations to be effective March 22, 1983.[119] Among other provisions, these regulations required conspicuous posting of notices in pediatric wards and nurseries advising that federal law prohibits a discriminatory failure to provide medical care to handicapped infants. The regulations also announced a toll-free HHS hot line to receive reports of discriminatory treatment; there was a promise of immediate investigation of all complaints. In the event of an investigation, institutions were required to provide federal investigators with access to facilities and with relevant medical records upon twenty-four hours notice.

Alarmed by the specter of federal investigators swooping into neonatal intensive care units and disrupting hospital routine, the American Academy of Pediatrics and the National Association of Children's Hospitals brought suit in federal court in the District of Columbia to prevent implementation of the HHS regulations. Virtually simultaneously, the American Hospital Association sued in the federal district court of New York in an effort to invalidate the HHS regulations. On April 14, 1983, within a month of the regulations' effective date, Judge Gesell in the federal district court in the District of Columbia declared the regulations to be invalid.[120] He ruled that HHS had failed to follow proper procedures in adopting the disputed regulations, as the agency had not allowed for prior notice to the public and a period of public comment on the proposed regulations. In addition, Judge Gesell held that the regulations were "arbitrary and capricious" in failing to consider that the hot line process might disrupt ongoing medical treatment, and that treatment might be inappropriate for an infant facing an unavoidable death. Judge Gesell did not determine whether, in principle, Section 504 of the Rehabilitation Act of 1973 could be applied to the issue of medical treatment for defective newborns.

HHS responded by correcting the procedural faults in the issuance of the Section 504 "Baby Doe" regulations, as they are sometimes called. On July 5, 1983, HHS published proposed regulations and requested public comment. In those proposed rules, HHS clarified that Section 504 would not be deemed applicable to "futile acts or therapies . . . which merely temporarily prolong the process of dying. . . ."[121] Otherwise, the Department's approach to Section 504 and the section's applicability to defective newborns remained unchanged. For example, HHS contended that a spina bifida child could not legally go untreated if the decision not to treat was grounded on the anticipated mental or physical impairment of the infant (as opposed to the futility of medical intervention to save the infant's life).

After the proposed regulations attracted over 16,000 comments, a slightly revised version of the July 1983 regulations was adopted by HHS on January 12, 1984.[122] The 1984 version required a smaller notice to be posted in hospitals, and provided that the notice need be posted only in areas accessible to hospital personnel rather than to parents or visitors. The new notice stated that federal law precluded withholding of "medically beneficial treatment" from handicapped infants solely on the basis of the infants' present or anticipated impairments. Interpretive guidelines explained that medical intervention could be withheld where it would clearly be futile and would only prolong the act of dying.[123] The 1984 version of the regulations provided both for federal intervention against suspected statutory violations, and for state intervention through efforts of state child protection agencies to compel life-preserving medical treatment for handicapped newborns. Those regulations also encouraged, but did not mandate, establishment of institutional child care review committees in hospitals.

The HHS "Baby Doe" regulations, both as originally and as finally adopted, drew sharp criticism on a variety of grounds. Some sources objected to direct federal intervention, which was viewed as usurping the traditional state and local role governing the responsibility of parents toward children. Others feared the zealousness of the prospective federal invaders. They saw federal investigations and seizure of medical records as disruptive of ongoing delivery of neonatal care. Additonally, some health care providers feared that the federal regulations would create an atmosphere of divisiveness or distrust among parents and medical staff, thus disrupting a trusting relation between parents and pediatric staff. Still other sources saw the federal standards as inherently vague, potentially prompting pediatric physicians to practice "defensive medicine" and to "overtreat" in order to avoid any suspicion of violating Section 504. It was feared that the Baby Doe regulations would prompt physicians to vigorously intervene to save infants who could not benefit from treatment, i.e., infants whose condition was so dismal that they ought to be permitted to expire.[124]

The fate of the HHS Baby Doe regulations adopted pursuant to Section 504 is in grave doubt as of this writing (September 1986). The American Hospital Association in early 1984, after publication of the final version of the HHS regulations, renewed its attack on those regulations in federal district court in New York contending that the regulations were not authorized by Congress in the Rehabilitation Act of 1973. That is, the Association asserted that individual medical decisions affecting defective newborns were not within the scope of services which Congress intended to reach in its 1973 anti-discrimination measure.

Federal courts in New York sustained this broad attack on the validity of the regulations.[125] The Second Circuit Court of Appeals ruled that Congress in adopting the Rehabilitation Act did not intend to encompass the matter of medical treatment decisions for defective newborns. That court viewed a 1973 Senate Report and 1977 HEW regulations referring to the Act's applicability to "health services" as intending to guarantee access to health care institutions, but not to govern medical treatment decisions. The court also noted that the relevant administrative agency (first HEW, then HHS) had not suggested between 1973 and 1982 that the Rehabilitation Act covered medical decisions for defective infants. Finally, the court was dubious that Congress intended to regulate such a delicate and complex matter as individual treatment decisions for handicapped infants, at least not without explicit Congressional consideration of the issue. In other settings, such as Medicare and Medicaid, Congress had generally avoided federal scrutiny of individual treatment decisions.

In June 1986, in a case called *Bowen v. American Hospital Association*, (106 S. Ct. 2101 [1986]. *Bowen* was a 5–3 decision, with 1 justice [Burger] concurring only in the judgment and not joining the plurality opinion for the Court) the U.S. Supreme Court took the teeth out of HHS' efforts to use Section 504 to become a federal watchdog over hospital practices relating to defective newborns. The Court ruled that the mandatory portions of the Baby Doe regulations (mainly parts ordering hospitals to post notices and ordering state child protection agencies to take steps to prevent medical neglect of defective infants) were not authorized by Congress in adopting the Rehabilitation Act of 1973. The key to the Supreme Court decision was a determination that the Act could only be applied (if at all) to hospital failures to treat defective newborns whose parents had authorized treatment. According to the Court, if the parents had not authorized treatment, a hospital's failure to treat would be prompted by lack of legal authority to override parental choice and not by "discrimination" against the handicapped as required by the Act. HHS had failed to present any evidence that in practice hospitals had refused to administer treatment authorized by an appropriate agency such as the parents. The mandatory HHS regulations did not, therefore, have a sufficient empirical base to justify their existence under Congress' anti-discrimination object.

By focusing the impact of Section 504 on instances where parents have otherwise authorized treatment for a newborn, the Supreme Court has certainly blunted HHS' drive to secure direct federal supervision of hospital practices in this area. For as the Court noted, hospitals do not commonly refuse treatment which parents have sought. Nonetheless, there are hints in *Bowen* that HHS might be able to revive its supervisory efforts by focusing on the advice given by personnel within hospitals to guide parents in making decisions on behalf of defective newborns. (However, the plurality opinion doubted that Section 504 could ever preclude hospital staff from recommending to the parents courses of action permitted by state law.) If HHS persists in its effort to utilize Section 504 in the context of handicapped newborns, it may eventually become necessary to resolve the issue decided negatively by the Second Circuit Court of Appeals but left open in *Bowen*—whether Section 504 can ever apply to individual medical decisions involving handicapped infants.

There are good policy reasons for not applying the Rehabilitation Act to neonatal treatment decisions in the absence of a more deliberately expressed Congressional intention.

The statutory definition of discrimination against the handicapped, with its reference to "otherwise qualified" persons, is rather opaque as applied to medical treatment for handicapped newborns. In other contexts in which Section 504 has been applied, the "otherwise qualified" language has been interpreted to mean that the handicap in question must be unrelated to the service to which access is sought by the handicapped individual.[126] This approach recognizes that there are some situations in which a handicap is in fact related to the affected individual's qualifications for the service being sought. For example, a blind person may not be suited for a nursing career and consequently may be legally excludable from a nurses' training program. As applied to medical treatment for defective newborns, this would apparently mean that situations might exist in which certain handicaps (and their related symptomatology) might be part of the basis for denying treatment for a newborn. The precise considerations and standards for their application have been, and still are, subjects of considerable dispute, as explained in the early sections of this chapter. Congress in 1973 gave no deliberation to this complex issue. And HHS, in stretching the Rehabilitation Act to apply, appears to have gone its own route in defining the statutory term "otherwise qualified" as applied to handicapped newborns. The final version of the HHS "Baby Doe" regulations appear to be heavy-handed, with little leeway for the kinds of considerations deemed relevant to decision-making under the "best interests of the infant" standard which has emerged in the state court decisions.

The interpretive guidelines issued by HHS as an appendix to the January 1984 Baby Doe regulations make clear that "medical benefit" is, according to the administering agency, the key to determining violations of Section 504.[127] The guidelines state that an infant who will (or even might) "medically benefit" from treatment is an "otherwise qualified" individual under Section 504. If treatment is then withheld "solely on the basis of present or anticipated physical or mental impairments," unlawful discrimination has taken place unless the hospital has taken steps to secure review of the nontreatment decision by an outside agency or court.

The illustrations offered by HHS to show "absence of medical benefit" indicate a somewhat narrow scope to that concept. For example, "futile treatment" is not considered to be of "medical benefit."[128] Futile treatment is then defined as treatment which will "temporarily prolong the act of dying of a terminally ill infant." The illustrations further explain that vigorous intervention might be omitted for a low birth weight infant based on a reasonable medical judgment of "improbability of success" or "risks of potential harm to the infant." But the kinds of "harm" deemed sufficient to omit treatment are not enumerated.

With the possible exception of the cryptic reference to "potential harm," HHS' intention appears to be to equate medical benefit with survival. That is, if an infant's life can be maintained beyond a short period of time, treatment would be deemed beneficial and would have to be administered. This position would be consistent with the current Surgeon General's announced position that an infant's life-preserving care can be omitted only when it would merely prolong a dying process, and not because the quality of prospective life is too dismal to be sustained.[129]

The HHS approach pursuant to section 504 was overly simplistic or heavy handed in its failure to acknowledge sufficiently a relation between certain impairments to infants and the soundness of vigorous medical intervention. The 1984 interpretive guidelines under Section 504 offer little or no leeway for the common medical practice of considering whether medical treatment will ultimately serve the best interests of the infant. Certain disabilities are clearly relevant to such a determination. For example, the mentation of a partial anencephalic may be so minimal that the infant—even if medically preservable for a substantial period—cannot reach a cognitive state which is a prerequisite to deriving human benefit from existence. Similarly, an infant's impairment may entail such unavoidable pain and suffering that preservation—even if possible for a long term—is not in that infant's best interests. An infant with Lesch-Nyhan syndrome—deranged and fated to engage in continuous self-mutilation—may offer an example.

It is conceivable that a legislature would exalt preservation of existence over consideration of prospective benefits and burdens for a defective newborn. But this was in no way what Congress did in adopting the Rehabilitation Act of 1973. That 1973 Congress did not deliberate about the complex and delicate issues involved in propounding treatment policies toward defective newborns. Congress did not then consider the emerging capacity of technology to preserve terribly debilitated infants who would formerly have perished despite all medical efforts. Congress did not consider the moral and ethical status of emerging medical practices of selective nontreatment (such as the practices regarding newborns with spina bifida). Moreover, when Congress did examine the issue of life-preserving care for defective newborns, in 1984, it adopted an approach which differs significantly from that adopted by HHS in its regulations under Section 504.

A divergence between the HHS Baby Doe regulations under Section 504 and Congress' 1984 amendments to the Child Abuse Prevention Act of 1978 furnishes an additional basis for finding the Baby Doe regulations to be totally unauthorized by the Rehabilitation Act of 1973. While some members of Congress argued that the 1984 child abuse amendments were "complimentary" to the HHS regulations,[130] analysis of the 1984 Amendments, as will be undertaken below, discloses some fundamental differences in the respective regulatory frameworks.

The 1984 Congress was intentionally noncommittal on the specific issue of whether the Rehabilitation Act of 1973 should be read to cover medical treatment of defective newborns. While Congress stated that nothing in the 1984 Act should be read to prejudice any existing rights under Section 504, this formulation was clearly intended as a "neutral" expression pending resolution of the issue by the courts.[131] In short, even without a clearcut Supreme Court declaration in *Bowen* that the Rehabilitation Act of 1973 does not reach individual medical decisions, it would make good sense for HHS to forego its reliance on Section 504, and to rely instead on Congress' policy toward defective newborns as expressed in the 1984 Amendments.

In the Child Abuse Amendments of 1984, [132] Congress spoke for the first time directly to the issue of withholding life-preserving medical treatment from defective infants. The general policy or spirit of the legislation was clearcut. An overwhelming majority of Congress opposed denial of "medically indicated treatment or nutrition" to disabled infants.[133] The 1982 Infant Doe case in Indiana was generally viewed by legislators as an abuse of parental prerogatives, a form of child abuse, and Congress was interested in curbing such abuses. The problem was how to further that end without needlessly disrupting ongoing processes of pediatric care.

Parts of the legislative program were totally unexceptional. For example, Congress decided to encourage formation of internal hospital committees to formulate institutional policies toward disabled infants, educate hospital personnel, and offer "counsel and review" of specific decisions regarding omission of life-preserving care.[134] This was fully consistent with the approach adopted by HHS in its Section 504 regulations, as described above. (Of course, because of the litigation described above, the fate of those HHS regulations was in doubt at the time that Congress adopted the 1984 amendments in question.) Another uncontroversial step by Congress was to promote operation of national and regional clearinghouses of information concerning medical treatment and community resources aiding disabled infants.[135] No one can dispute that treatment decisions ought to be well informed, including full information about the medical and social resources available.

A significant departure under the 1984 Amendments was a Congressional effort to compel state child protection agencies to establish processes for preventing medical neglect of disabled infants. In order to qualify for federal grants relating to child abuse prevention (and it was anticipated that every state would desire to so qualify), state child protection services were required to adopt procedures to promote reporting, investigation, and legal intervention in possible cases of medical neglect of disabled infants. The processes adopted by the states would have to include hospital designation of a person to whom personnel could report suspected cases of infant medical neglect, notification of the state child protection agency by such a designated individual in the case of suspected neglect, and agency authority to pursue legal remedies to prevent implementation of treatment choices deemed to constitute neglect.[136]

The invocation of state child neglect agencies in the context of defective newborns was not entirely novel. The disputed HHS regulations pursuant to Section 504 had also sought to enlist state agencies in preventing the withholding of medically indicated treatment from disabled infants. A departure in the 1984 Amendments was Congressional willingness to rely primarily (and perhaps exclusively) on state and local machinery to prevent medical neglect of defective newborns. Several principal sponsors of the legislation emphasized that *federal* intervention was *not* anticipated under the scheme being adopted.[137] By contrast, HHS had been employing federal investigations regularly in its administration of regulations pursuant to Section 504.[138] The return of principal responsibility to the state agencies was apparently viewed both by federal legislators and affected health care providers as a positive step. There had been widespread apprehension about roving federal "Baby Doe" squads intervening in pediatric units, a specter viewed as an ultimate manifestation of the federal government as "Big Brother."

Perhaps the most critical element of the 1984 Amendments was the statutory definition provided for the term "withholding of medically indicated treatment"—the key to the definition of the medical neglect that state child protection agencies were being assigned to prevent. That is, every state desiring to secure federal funds relating to child abuse protection programs would have to show that the state's legal apparatus was aligned to prevent "withholding of medically indicated treatment" from defective newborns. According to Congress, this key term meant "failure to respond to the infant's life-threatening conditions" by not providing treatment which in the treating physician's "reasonable medical judgment [would] be most likely to be effective in ameliorating or correcting all such [life-threatening] conditions."[139] However, there were three exceptions listed to the statutory mandate of vigorous medical intervention. Treatment (other than "appropriate nutrition, hydration, or medication") could be foregone where, in the physician's reasonable medical judgment: a) the infant is irreversibly comatose; b) treatment would merely prolong dying or otherwise "be futile in terms of the survival of the infant"; or c) such treatment would be "virtually futile" in terms of survival and the treatment would be "inhumane."

This definition of medically indicated treatment—with its explicit reference to physicians' medical judgment and its provision for three exceptions to an obligation to continue life-preserving treatment—enjoyed widespread support. The language had been hammered out in negotiations among Senate staff and representatives of a number of interested groups. The groups reflected interests of health care providers, disabled citizens, and right to life advocates. Among the groups who endorsed the final definition were the American Hospital Association, the American Academy of Pediatrics, the National Association of Children's Hospitals, the American Nurses' Association, the Association for Retarded Citizens, the Spina Bifida Association of America, and the National Right to Life Committee.[140] Though the American Medical Association was opposed, the legislation was adopted by overwhelming margins in both the Senate and in the House.

This apparent concensus on a volatile issue is all the more surprising because some of the groups eventually supportive were originally staunchly opposed to any government intrusion into neonatal units. Moreover, in both houses of the Congress, some speakers had lamented government interference in what they considered an intimate family decision to be made in consultation with medical staff.[141] In the House of Representatives, an effort had been made to remove all provisions relating to enforcement of child neglect laws against parental nontreatment decisions and to simply encourage advisory committees to be established within institutions to assist sound decision-making concerning defective newborns.[142] The effort was repulsed by a vote of 231 to 182.

In light of the surprising compromise among divergent groups, the ultimate impact of the 1984 Amendments on ongoing medical practices and on the administration of state child neglect statutes is hard to gauge. Groups such as the American Hospital Association and the American Academy of Pediatrics obviously thought that they could live with the definition of "medically indicated treatment" as adopted. Perhaps they were relying on the deference to "reasonable medical judgment" contained in the statutory language and were assuming that the medical judgment provision would sufficiently insulate physicians' customary decisions against overly intrusive scrutiny. Yet the "judgment" accorded to physicians by the statute is confined to specific issues—to the effectiveness of proposed treatments and to the presence of one of the three exceptions to the normal obligation to administer life-preserving treatment. The first two exceptions—for comatose infants and for terminally ill infants whose survival can't be secured—are indeed salutary concessions to the direction in which sound neonatal care had moved. But these two provisions provide only part of the necessary leeway. The third exception—for treatment which would be both "virtually futile in terms of the survival of the infant" and "inhumane"—might be read as too narrow to accommodate sound medical practice as it has emerged under the rubric of "best interests of the infant."[143]

The real impact of the 1984 Amendments upon medical practice remains speculative. In December 1984, HHS published "proposed regulations" to implement the 1984 Amendments. Those regulations, if adopted, would have greatly constricted medical flexibility by giving a narrow interpretation to the statutory "exceptions" to the concept of mandatory "medically indicated treatment."[144] For example, as to the exception for "futile" treatment which would "merely prolong dying," HHS contended that treatment could be withheld only if an infant's death was "imminent" (as opposed to a terminal condition which would become immediately life-threatening in the future).[145] As to the exception for "virtually futile treatment" which would be "inhumane," the proposed regulations sought to impose two limitations. First, HHS defined "virtually futile" as meaning a situation where "treatment is highly unlikely to prevent *imminent* death."[146] Second, "inhumane" was confined to situations where the proposed treatment by itself would produce pain and suffering or other medical contraindications (such as paralysis) which would make the treatment inhumane.[147]

In response to the proposed regulations, HHS received 116,000 letters, including a letter from six key legislators who had sponsored the 1984 amendments and had helped to hammer out its "compromise" language. This letter from Congressional sponsors chiefly criticized HHS' use of the term "imminent" to define the time period between contemplated treatment and a death which would render the treatment "futile."[148] The letter explained that "imminence" was a problematic term (particularly in light of medical uncertainty about the proximity of death) and that the term had intentionally been dropped from the legislation. Several medical and hospital organizations also criticized the definitions that had been formulated in HHS' proposed regulations, primarily on the basis that medical judgment had been too severely confined by the definitions.

In its final regulations adopted in April 1985, HHS backtracked considerably. With regard to interpretation of the key term "withholding of medically indicated treatment," the Department let the statutory language speak for itself without any "clarifying definitions." "Interpretive guidelines" were issued, but were relegated to an appendix which was specifically deemed not to constitute a binding rule of law.[149]

Those April 1985 interpretive guidelines also retreated somewhat from the positions adopted by HHS in its proposed regulations of

December 1984. For example, in response to the letter from the six legislators, the term imminent was deleted with regard to both futile and virtually futile treatment. The Department continued to insist, though, in its nonbinding appendix that life-preserving treatment could not be withheld as futile if the unavoidable death would occur "in the more distant future," meaning several years hence.[150] Moreover, HHS maintained that where treatment is deemed virtually futile because of the very slight chance of ultimately salvaging the infant, a further finding that treatment would be "inhumane" hinges on assessment of negative factors (pain, suffering, and other contraindications such as organic damage) flowing exclusively from the treatment itself.[151]

The actual Congressional intent is not easy to gauge. The "virtually futile" and "inhumane" language did not draw much attention in the Congressional debates. An "explanatory statement" by six key sponsors of the relevant Senate bill does not shed much light. It merely points out that humaneness is not excluded elsewhere in the language defining "medically indicated treatment" just because the term inhumane is explicitly mentioned in the context of "virtually futile" treatment.[152] The six sponsors then mention that humaneness is a factor to be considered "in selecting among effective treatments." This reference to effective treatments seem cryptic in the context of a clause addressing "virtually futile" treatments.

One interpretation of the critical language was provided by a sponsor of the Senate bill, Senator Nickles. He asserted that the "virtually futile" exception covered a gray area where the infant has only a slim chance of survival and the physician must make "a judgment call as to whether the odds of correcting the child's condition are strong enough to merit an attempt to save the baby, even with treatment that may be very painful."[153] This interpretation jibes with the statutory language but, if accurate, seems to leave a discontinuity between Congress' definition of required "medically indicated treatment" and the standard of "best interests of the infant" previously endorsed in judicial decisions and in position statements by important medical providers such as the AMA and the American Academy of Pediatrics.[154]

The HHS suggestion that "inhumane" treatment (in the context of virtually futile therapy) should be determined exclusively according to consequences of the treatment itself (i.e., by consideration of potential iatrogenic conditions), provides a highly unnatural and unfortunate perspective. According to this perspective, in considering the prospective suffering of an infant patient the decision-maker is supposed to distinguish between suffering produced by the existing pathological conditions and suffering to be produced by the proposed treatment.

The former type of suffering apparently isn't supposed to count. Such an approach seems both physically impossible to implement and absurd. If a very low birth weight infant suffers from paroxysms of cough and breathing difficulties associated with underdeveloped lungs, a question might exist as to whether to perform a tracheotomy to facilitate breathing. In making a decision, the HHS approach would focus attention on additional pain, discomfort, or risks associated with the proposed treatment (tracheotomy), but would ignore the continuous pain or suffering associated with the underdeveloped lungs and other organs. Similarly, in the case of a spina bifida infant, HHS focus would be on added suffering or risk connected with closing the spinal sac or installing a shunt, in disregard of pain or discomfort associated with the underlying conditions of paralysis, incontinence, etc. Good medical judgment, which the HHS purports to support, would not tolerate such distinctions among sources of suffering in deciding what is humane or inhumane.

A key question pursuant to the 1984 Amendments is whether required "medically indicated treatment" encompasses situations in which an infant's life can be extended for a considerable period, but at a cost of such suffering and limited function that it would be in the infant's best interests to forego life-preserving medical intervention. The issue arises, for example, regarding some spina bifida cases with high lesions (making very severe disabilities likely) who could be preserved for at least a number of years if aggressive medical intervention were undertaken. If the infant's prospective life entails net burdens rather than benefits (using a calculus which excludes social worth considerations or burdens on others), then vigorous treatment leading to protracted preservation is counter to the infant's best interests, and may even be cruel.

Perhaps the withholding of surgical intervention from some spina bifida infants can be reconciled with the statutory language by saying that the pathological condition (exposed spinal sac and accompanying disabilities) is not immediately life-threatening. This would be along the lines of the approach taken by the New York courts in *Baby Jane Doe* in endorsing conservative medical treatment, meaning antibiotics, but not surgery to close the open wound. Indeed, the statutory language tends to support this approach; for the definition of medical neglect (failure to provide "medically indicated treatment") is confined to failure to treat "life-threatening conditions." However, many physicians would, in extremely severe cases of spina bifida, recommend that antibiotics be omitted in the expectation that an infection would set in and the infant would be permitted to die. At least at the time of the infection, the infant would be suffering from a life-threatening condition and the statutory language about medical neglect would become relevant.

Perhaps the statutory mention of "inhumane" treatment (along with "virtually futile") in the third exception to required treatment will suffice to allow net long-term benefits and burdens to come into play. That is, the "inhumane" concept could conceivably be the handle through which the "best interests of the infant" formula is incorporated into the framework of the 1984 Amendments. This is especially so in light of the mention by Congressional sponsors of the 1984 Amendments that consideration of "inhumane" intervention is not to be confined to the statutory clause relating to "virtually futile" treatment.[155] Concepts of humane handling are therefore also relevant in making a "reasonable medical judgment" whether treatment will likely be "effective in ameliorating or correcting" all life-threatening conditions. If spina bifida, with its associated impairments, is regarded as the life-threatening condition, then a physician might conscientiously make a judgment in severe cases that no treatment would be "effective" in "ameliorating or correcting" the condition. But if the life-threatening condition is regarded as an infection which subsequently sets in, then antibiotic treatment will certainly "ameliorate" the condition.

In sum, the statutory language is not very felicitous in promoting the best interests of the disabled infant as part of the medical neglect definition. The conjunction of "inhumane" with "virtually futile" is liable to prompt an interpretation of medical neglect in which the infant's prospective suffering is weighed by decision-makers only where the chances of an extended period of survival are very slim. This would be contrary to the judicial trend to accord deference to a conscientious parental judgment (made in conjunction with medical personnel) that further treatment would be contrary to the best interests of a severely defective infant even in some situations in which long-term survival is attainable with vigorous intervention. I'll comment further on this aspect of the 1985 HHS regulations in the last chapter, "On Death and the Quality of Life."

Professor Thomas Murray has predicted that the 1985 HHS regulations "will have little or no effect on current practices"[156] He points out that even if the Department's suggested guidelines were enforced by HHS, the practical consequences would be modest. That is, the ultimate federal sanction for state noncompliance is disqualification from access to a rather small amount of federal aid relating to child abuse prevention programs. (Indeed, the relevant total available for *all* states for fiscal year 1985 was in the range of $12 million.[157]) Professor Murray also points to the reaction of the president of the American Academy of Pediatricians who in April 1985 issued a press release hailing the HHS final regulations as reaffirming "the role of reasonable medical judgment and [reaffirming] that decisions should be made in the best interests of the infant."[158] Presumably, this can be taken as some indication that practitioners will not see their current practices as impeded by the 1984 federal legislation.

The psychological impact of the HHS "interpretive guidelines" might be significantly greater than their slight legal force. HHS anticipated that all states would be interested in applying for child abuse prevention grants and therefore that all states would be interested in complying with the federal conditions. While the 1985 appendix is explicitly deemed nonbinding, the interpretive guidelines would not have been issued unless it was thought that they would have some impact.[159] Some states may be very willing to follow the federal suggestions; indeed, at least some state legislative movement in the direction of the HHS positions has already been signalled.[160] At the very least, the widely publicized HHS efforts may impact on medical practice simply by setting a tone which encourages overly aggressive medical intervention in handling defective newborns.

Another possible regression accomplished by the 1984 amendments is the ostensible prohibition on withholding of nutrition from defective newborns. Under the statutory definition of "medically indicated treatment," appropriate nutrition may not be withheld even when medical treatment would merely prolong dying. The intendment of appropriate nutrition is not explained. I fear that the intention was to preclude withholding of nutrition in virtually all situations.[161] This broad prohibition might be proper as regards oral feeding of a patient capable of ingesting and digesting food. But the ban is misplaced as applied to artificial feeding. Recent cases dealing with incompetent adult patients have made clear that at least in the context of a terminally ill patient, artificial nutrition can be regarded as a form of medical treatment and withheld according to the same criteria applicable to withholding of treatment generally. I will argue at the end of this chapter that a similar approach ought to be applied to infant patients. In some instances it is humane, a net relief of suffering, to withhold artificial nutrition from a severely defective and dying newborn. Hopefully, child protection service agencies will concur that continued artificial feeding is not appropriate nutrition in such instances.

State Statutes

At least three states—Arizona, Indiana, and Louisiana—have within recent years amended their legislation dealing with child neglect to explicitly prohibit the denial of medical treatment or of nutrition to some handicapped newborns. This legislation reflects some unhappiness with the increasingly publicized phenomenon of withholding medical intervention from infants born with physical and mental impairments.

The two most detailed legislative provisions were adopted in Louisiana, in 1982, and Arizona, in 1983 (with amendments in 1984). The Louisiana measure goes the furthest in restricting the situations in which life-preserving medical treatment can legally be withheld from a defective infant. The Louisiana statute forbids withholding from any infant medical care which is necessary (according to competent medical judgment) to save the life of the infant. The statutory prohibition is specifically made applicable "despite the opinion of the child's parent or parents, the physician, or others that the quality of the child's life would be deficient should the child live."[162] Exceptions are provided only for a child in a permanently comatose state, or for situations where "the potential risks to the child's life or health inherent in the treatment or surgery itself outweigh the potential benefits for survival from the treatment or surgery itself."[163] This last exception was ostensibly intended to cover iatrogenic conditions, instances when the prospective medical procedures would seriously risk brain damage, or increased paralysis, or the like. In addition, the Louisiana legislature banned deprivation of food, water, nutrients, or oxygen from an infant for any reason.[164]

The 1984 Arizona legislation, while similar in some respects to Louisiana's is somewhat more flexible in providing leeway to decision-makers on behalf of defective newborns to withhold life-preserving treatment. As in Louisiana, the Arizona statute is aimed at deprivation of "necessary lifesaving medical treatment or surgical care."[165] But there are several parts of the statute which mitigate this broad prohibition. First, the legislation explicitly provides that in assessing medical necessity, "reasonable medical judgments" among alternative courses of treatment shall be respected.[166] Furthermore, there are statutory exceptions broader than those in Louisiana. Arizona picks up on the originally proposed HHS regulations by exempting "futile treatment or treatment that will do no more than prolong the act of dying when death is imminent."[167] An exemption is also provided where "the potential risk to the infant's life or health . . . outweighs the potential benefit to the infant of the treatment or care."[168] Significantly, the potential risks to be considered in the weighing process are not limited to those inherent in the treatment or surgery itself, as was the case in Louisiana. Nor is there condemnatory reference in Arizona's statutory scheme to "quality of life" opinions, as was the case in Louisiana. Finally, Arizona legislation differs from Louisiana in promoting infant care review committees in hospitals in order to assist institutions in complying with the standards of neonatal care described above.[169] (Like Louisiana, however, Arizona does ban denial of "nourishment" from a newborn infant "for any reason."[170])

Indiana also adopted legislation (in 1983) aimed in part at confining the situations in which handicapped newborns are deprived of life-preserving medical treatment. Indiana provided that neglected children—on whose behalf state child protection agency intervention is available—will include handicapped children deprived of treatment "necessary to remedy or ameliorate a life threatening medical condition, if the nutrition or medical or surgical intervention is generally provided to similarly situated handicapped or nonhandicapped children."[171]

None of the recent state legislative schemes has as yet been definitively interpreted. A key question is whether these measures permit parents, acting in conjunction with medical personnel, to withhold medical treatment on the basis that the defective infant's prospective physical and emotional suffering outweigh any benefits of prospective existence. The answer would appear to be "no" with regard to Louisiana, where the legislature specifically banned decisions grounded on the quality of an infant's prospective life. The answer in Arizona and Indiana is less clear. The Indiana language is inherently vague on the matter, because it doesn't speak to whether prospective suffering is a basis for differentiating certain defective newborns from "similarly situated" infants. In Arizona, the critical question is whether "potential risks to life or health" (to be considered against potential benefits) can include the prospective pain and suffering of a severely defective infant flowing from his original impairments, as opposed to impairments accompanying iatrogenic conditions caused by medical intervention. As noted above, there are some oblique indications from the statutory language—when contrasted with the more detailed Louisiana language—that the answer will be positive, in other words, that the suffering from the defective infant's original impairments may be weighed. For example, Arizona did not restrict the "risks" to be considered to those "inherent" in the medical or surgical procedures themselves. If the answer is in fact positive, the statute would, in effect, allow decision-makers to operate according to the judicially evolved "best interests of the infant" standard.

Some commentators argue that broad legislation on the matter of withholding life-preserving treatment from defective newborns is premature. Their contention is that the issue is too nuanced or complex for reduction to a statutory formula. According to this view, the variables in decision-making are multiple, and the social values and priorities still in flux, so that parents and medical staff should be permitted to "muddle through" in their anguishing decisions, pending the emergence of greater societal concensus.[172]

Because there have been no definitive interpretations of the legislative efforts to date, either on the state or federal plane, assessment of the legislative route may be premature. But certain general observations can be offered. First, legislation does have the potential for quickly removing what has been a pervasive uncertainty about the scope of permissible decisions to withhold life-preserving care from defective infants, as well as for promoting consistency of decision-making over diverse geographical areas (at least on a statewide basis). Second, legislative bodies have the capacity, and perhaps the duty, to fix basic parameters of decision-making in accord with social conscience. Issues such as the relevance of economic costs to decision-making, the inclusion of parents and sibling interests in decision-making, or the prerogative of parents to surrender responsibility for raising a defective child are all subject to legislative resolution. For example, the recent federal legislative guidelines authorizing omission of "futile" or "virtually futile" care help instruct medical personnel that not every infant must be vigorously maintained, at least when duration of an infant's prospective existence is limited. Moreover, legislatures certainly have a potential role in allocating sufficient societal resources to assure that impaired infants are not relegated to inhuman conditions after their lives are preserved.

The notion that if legislatures simply keep "hands off," parental discretion and medical judgment will be allowed to fix appropriate parameters, seems misguided. Even if legislatures did not change the statutory status quo, the courts would inevitably confront the issue of authority to withdraw life-preserving care in the context of existing general child neglect and abuse statutes (even if those statutes were not amended to explicitly cover defective newborns). And no court has been willing to interpret such statutes as affording parents a prerogative—even under the rubric of "family privacy"—to do more than make decisions guided by the best interests of the infant as the predominant standard. The judiciary would then have to make the same kinds of value choices— about parental and sibling interests, and about allocation of resources— as the legislative bodies must face in outlining the parameters of parental decision-making.

The primary danger from legislative action seems to be that legislators, operating in the context of political pressures from extreme right-to-life advocates, will overreact against some past abuses and will end up restricting sound and humane decision-making. The judicially evolved "best interests of the infant" standard remains the best overall guide and ought not to be eliminated. As noted, legislatures can resolve some of the hard questions relating to the precise meaning of "best interests"—such as the relevance of sibling interests or parental economic burdens—but the best interests standard ought to remain the predominant guide.

Abuses can be corralled under the best interests rubric without disrupting sensitive decison-making. As in the context of adult patients facing life-threatening conditions, it is important to recognize that mitigation of suffering is an interest that can coexist with, and must enjoy equal status with, society's determination to promote respect for the value of human existence.

Infants and Starvation

Sometimes an infant born with multiple anomalies also suffers from a blockage or defect in the esophagus or gastrointestinal tract. If a determination is then made not to operate to correct the feeding blockage, and also not to provide parenteral nutrition, the consequence is that the infant will starve to death. This course has been followed in a number of reported instances, including the Johns Hopkins infant in 1961 and Infant Doe in 1982.

As in the case of adult patients, a serious question arises as to whether nutrition can be regarded as a form of medical intervention and can be withheld according to the criteria applicable to other forms of medical intervention. The emotional hurdle involved with starvation of an infant as a form of medical practice is even greater than in the case of adults. For the spectre of a fledgling, helpless being struggling for existence and being denied elementary sustenance normally provided is indeed heartrending. Moreover, a process of starvation may involve pain and physiological changes which are repulsive and distressing to surrounding medical personnel.[173] These factors prompted at least two states to entirely ban withholding of nutrition from infants, and prompted the Congressional admonition in the 1984 Child Care Amendments that "appropriate nutrition" should always be provided in the handling of newborns.

This leaves the question of when (and if) nutrition can be deemed inappropriate. Despite the emotional hurdles concerning the handling of newborns, the issue of artificial nutrition in this context ought to be resolved essentially in the same manner as in the case of adult patients. That is, if the basic criterion of best interests of the infant dictates the withholding of life-preserving medical intervention, artificial nutrition ought to be withholdable, so long as such a course would be humane. "Humaneness" in such an instance would entail consideration of the extent of irremediable pain and discomfort accompanying a starvation process, versus the net pain and discomfort ensuing if nutrition is maintained. As in the case of adult patients, personal scruples of medical personnel are relevant in the sense that no medical worker should be forced to participate in a course of handling as to which he or she is conscientiously opposed.

The soundness of this position—that withholding of artificial nutrition may be an acceptable medical option—is most evident where the obstacle to normal nutrition is itself a life-threatening anomaly. This is so, for example, in the case of an infant born with gastroschisis, the absence of a functioning intestine. Parenteral nutrition is possible for some period, but the ultimate death of the infant is unavoidable. If the net suffering of the infant (the suffering from the underlying anomaly discounted by any suffering which would accompany starvation) appears to outweigh any gains during the inexorable dying process, then the withholding of parenteral nutrition would seem to be the humane course. The status of the infant in this situation is comparable to that of the incompetent, inexorably dying adult patient whose palliative treatment is shaped by consideration of best interests, meaning net assessment of burdens and benefits. Numerous commentators have noted that there is little moral distinction between withholding artificial nutrition and withholding other forms of medical care in all such instances.[174]

The much harder question involves an infant with crippling deformities and multiple anomalies who does not face any rapidly lethal lesions and can survive for a protracted period of months or even years. If there were a fortuitously associated anomaly which prevented feeding, such as an intestinal atresia, the infant might well be permitted to expire from starvation without surgical intervention. Such a decision would be appropriate if application of the best interests standard would so indicate. But what if no atresia or other anomaly prevents feeding? Should the infant be permitted to starve if the weighing of net burdens and benefits seems to indicate that the infant would be better off dead than alive?

The resolution of this issue would seem to parallel the resolution of the nutrition issue in the context of incompetent adult patients.[175] There is an insurmountable revulsion toward withholding manual feeding from a being whose digestive system is functional and who seeks food. But when some naturally occurring defect exists which permits nutrition only through artificial medical means—whether through tubes, surgery, or injections—medical intervention to provide nutrition should be governed by the same criteria applicable to other medical care. That is, artificial nutrition can then be omitted (and palliative care such as analgesics administered) if the patient's conditions and prospects are so dismal that it is in that patient's own best interests to be permitted to die. Such a course is most natural when a patient is terminally ill and faces an inexorable dying process. But I have argued that such a course ought also to be available in rare instances where the patient is preservable for

some substantial period, but at an intolerable cost in physical and emotional suffering. As noted, any unrelievable pain associated with a starvation process would become a factor to be considered in weighing the best
interests of the infant.

The above distinction between artificial and natural feeding is not a
completely logical distinction. It might be that an infant being manually
fed would be better off dead than alive, and that an infant in a neighboring crib with identical prognosis will be allowed to expire because there is
some natural defect present which makes artificial feeding necessary.
But this situation is not markedly different from that of neighboring
adult hospital patients in the same degree of deterioration, when one of
them is allowed to expire without antibiotics upon the fortuitous onset of
pneumonia or is allowed to expire from a heart attack without artificial
resuscitation, while the other patient lingers in an indefinite deteriorated
state.

The differentiations here are dictated by important emotional and
psychological factors. American society is not willing to endorse withholding of manual feeding from beings who are capable and desirous of
swallowing and digesting food. When natural illness occurs, and becomes life-threatening, we are willing to "let nature take its course"—
including withholding of artificial nutrition—so long as the best interests
of the incompetent patient so dictate.

Logic is not the only factor in this setting. It is arguable that the *most*
"humane" course would be to administer a merciful injection (active
euthanasia) in order to spare the infant whatever suffering is attendant
upon a starvation process despite sedation. But American society will not
endorse active administration of death, even for the terminally ill and
suffering. And so long as reasonably humane results are attainable
through passively withholding medical intervention according to the
best interests of incompetent patients, that is probably the best course.
Authorization of active euthanasia would entail revision of the criminal
law in every jurisdiction, and would significantly alter the popular perception of a physician's role. Society has adjusted (or is adjusting) to the
notion that when the physician can't heal, easing of the natural dying
process is appropriate. It may be true that there is little moral or practical difference between pulling a plug on a respirator in order to allow a
patient to pass away and administering an injection of curare. Nonetheless, if society is comfortable with this line, and if humane results are
attainable through "passive" handling (including the termination of previously instituted medical treatment), then the system "ain't broke" and
ought not to be repaired.

VII

Afterword: On Death and the Quality of Life

In the appendix to the 1985 regulations implementing the Child Care Amendments of 1984, the following language appears concerning the import of Congress' definition of the "medically indicated treatment" which is intended to be mandatory in handling infants:

> [Statutory] focus on the potential effectiveness of treatment in ameliorating or correcting life-threatening conditions makes clear that it does not sanction decisions based on subjective opinions about the future 'quality of life' of a retarded or disabled person.[1]

This statement was welcomed by right to life groups as representing a great victory. In their eyes, it signalled federal disqualification of quality of life considerations from the context of medical handling of defective infants.

Their celebration seems misplaced. I very much doubt that the import of the 1984 Child Care Amendments is to eliminate "quality of life" considerations in the broad sense intended by the right to life organizations. Even skipping over the fact that the quoted language appears in a nonbinding appendix, the thrust of the HHS statement cannot be taken nearly as far as these organizations would like.

If the import of the HHS language is to disqualify social worth considerations from the context of life-preserving medical decisions, that step had long ago been accomplished. No American court or commentator has ever endorsed the notion that in the medical decision-making context an incompetent patient might be relinquished because the patient is not "worthy" of being preserved. To the contrary, decisions such as *Conroy* and *Saikewicz* have taken great pains to rule out such eugenic-like elements. I have suggested that the monmouth expense associated with some forms of treatment is a lurking omnipresence in medical decision-making, even if not an explicitly legitimated factor. But I doubt that any source, federal or otherwise, can eliminate that economic factor entirely from the decision-making context.

If the import of the HHS language is to disqualify stereotyped notions about the nature of a handicapped existence, the HHS admonition is useful (though it does not thereby eliminate quality of life considerations from the decision-making calculus). Subjective opinions which automatically equate a handicapped existence with unbearable frustration, helplessness, or worthlessness are indeed out of place in this context. Health care providers and parents making life or death determinations probably do need to be reminded that special resources are available to help handicapped persons cope and that the vast majority of handicapped persons cope in a fashion that makes their lives worthwhile to them.

If the intended thrust of the HHS language is to disqualify consideration of prospective pain and suffering from the decision-making formula, I doubt that the effort is either well considered or successful. There may be no place for facile assumptions about pain, but there must be room for consideration of suffering in determining an infant's fate. Virtually every observer concedes that some infants suffer terribly in their impaired state and that the suffering may reach levels where death is a welcome relief.[2] Humane handling in such an instance dictates withholding life-preserving medical intervention.

There is no question that the determination of when the burdens of existence outweigh the benefits is a delicate one. This helps explain the reluctance of most courts to accept the tort claim of a wrongful life cause of action (an attempt to collect damages for having been born, such as for a child who is born gravely defective after a negligent amniocentesis examination of the pregnant mother failed to detect the defect).[3] But the difficulty of the assessment of net prospective burdens and benefits for a defective infant ought not to prevent the humane course in those instances when it can be said in good conscience that the infant will be better off dead than alive.

Even given their most stringent interpretation, the Child Care Amendments of 1984 acknowledge the relevance of quality of life (meaning prospective suffering) in some instances. For the statute certainly establishes that medical intervention may be omitted for infants where it would be "futile" or "virtually futile" (meaning that survival is highly unlikely) and treatment would be "inhumane."[4] Even if inhumane is determined only according to factors flowing from iatrogenic conditions (increased paralysis, brain damage, or other contraindications), a reading which I vigorously oppose, the statute thus admits that quality of life factors such as suffering and additional disfunction can sometimes prompt a decision not to administer treatment to a defective newborn. Treatment which is destined to be "futile" might be capable of sustaining an infant's life for some brief span, and yet under the statutory language it can be foregone because it is understood that in some circumstances keeping the infant alive is inhumane. Similarly, if the treatment is virtually futile, meaning highly unlikely to secure survival, it may be foregone if it is judged "inhumane" in terms of contraindications. This recognizes that even though survival is *possible* (though unlikely) treatment might be unwarranted because of the negative consequences (suffering or increased disability) for the patient. In short, preservation of life is not deemed *the* supreme value to be furthered at any cost. Avoidance of pain, suffering, and extraordinary disfunction are legitimate concerns. Quality of life can thus be considered, at least in some circumstances.

As discussed in chapter 6, the import of the 1984 Amendments is harder to gauge with regard to infants born with disabilities that foretell an extremely disfunctional, though protractable, existence. Spina bifida children with high lesions and accompanying complications offer a prototype. The irresolution is understandable because the dilemma is excruciating. A handicapped life (like any other life) is ordinarily to be preserved with all means at hand; yet there are extremes at which vigorous medical intervention becomes inhumane from the perspective of the infant whose life is at stake. It can probably be said in good conscience that an infant who will spend its entire existence in total immobility, unable or barely able to relate to its environment, subject to repeated physical invasions (from surgery, shunts, tubes, etc.), and dependent on outside aid for every bodily function is suffering and is better off dead than alive. Then, the option of withholding life-preserving medical intervention ought to be available.

The main problems are medical predictability (for ultimate levels of disability may be hard to assess early on), and human capacity to appraise the feelings of a totally uncommunicative being with no prior life history to guide assessment of that being's wants or needs. I hesitantly conclude that there are conditions which entail such probable suffering and degradation that withholding of treatment is warranted even though existence could be preserved for years through maximum medical intervention. I can understand a contrary position which argues that either the elements which would warrant such terminal decisions are not measurable, or that we cannot trust parents and attending physicians to confine themselves to the appropriate criteria. Infant care review committees should therefore be installed to monitor such terminal decisions in order to ensure that humane considerations are indeed the moving forces.

In 1976, at an early juncture in the debate on the medical handling of defective newborns, an interdisciplinary group convened to formulate relevant guidelines. Among the tentative principles which emerged were the following:

> 1) every newborn has a moral value;
> 2) parents bear primary responsibility for the well-being of their off-spring;
> 3) physicians have a duty to employ medical measures conducive to the well-being of an infant;
> 4) the state has an interest in the proper fulfillment of the above responsibilities and duties regarding the well-being of an infant;
> 5) life-preserving intervention does harm (and can be omitted) where an infant cannot survive infancy, or will live in intractable pain, or "cannot participate even minimally in human experience."[5]

Those propositions are as sound today as when written; no formulation which I have seen surpasses them.

The pervasiveness of quality of life considerations—meaning suffering and dignity of the affected individual—is both more evident and more understandable in the context of competent adult medical patients. American law is moving more and more toward recognizing individual autonomy to direct medical intervention in the dying process. Particularly where death is unavoidable and lurking in the near future, an individual can fix the level of his or her medical care according to personal preferences regarding pain, dignity, and emotional suffering. A competent individual can decide what level of physical pain is tolerable and which elements of emotional suffering—including helplessness, dependence, embarrassment, and frustration at incapacity—dictate a cessation of life-preserving medical care. If the competent individual makes a clear expression of such preferences, that expression will be respected and implemented even after the individual loses capacity to make his or her own medical decisions.

It is becoming increasingly clear that this prerogative to shape the dying process ought not be confined to situations where death is imminent. Uncertainty of medical prediction, and recognition that suffering and indignity can be acutely felt over a protracted period (not just at the period when death is imminent), dictate such a result. Thus, a competent patient ought to be able to shape medical intervention where an inexorable dying process has begun.

Self-determination and liberty to resist bodily invasion may even be sufficiently strong societal interests to allow an individual to resist life-*saving* medical interventions—that is, medical interventions capable

of arresting the dying process and restoring the individual to a protracted existence. There are at least two kinds of situations in which
individual autonomy has been extended to this extreme. In the first
situation, religious precepts compel a person to resist life-saving treatment. In the second, quality of life considerations, such as distaste for an
extremely disabled existence, have prompted individuals to resist life-
saving amputations or long-term dialysis treatment. To my mind, deference accorded to individual autonomy in such instances does not undermine traditional societal concern for life as a sacrosanct value—any more
than the conduct of just wars does. In the latter instance, respect for life
is tempered by values of justice and patriotism. In the former case,
respect for life is tempered by values of self-determination, autonomy,
and bodily integrity. (For reconciliation of this position with traditional
governmental efforts to prevent suicide, see chapter 2, supra.)

Even in the context of incompetent dying patients, quality of life
elements have a limited, but appropriate place. In the face of an irreversible terminal condition, it is appropriate to ease the dying process of an
incompetent individual by withholding or withdrawing life-extending
treatment in order to ease suffering and preserve the individual's human
dignity. Subject to caveats about the difficulty of measuring pain or
pleasure in a near insensate patient, the object of relieving physical and
emotional suffering already enjoys widespread support. But when notions of human dignity are activated in order to justify a terminal result,
there will have to be broad societal concensus that the dying individual's
status is indeed so degrading (in light of the individual's prior vigor) that
permitting death is a "humane" gesture. Crystallization of the relevant
norms and standards of human dignity is still in its incipient stages.

The truly hard case—and the one that is most unresolved in the
jurisprudence—is where a marginal existence is preservable for an extended period. The focus here is the formerly competent and healthy
individual who has now deteriorated—usually because of chronic illness—to a level of complete physical helplessness and mental disfunction. The question is whether (in the absence of prior instructions from
the individual involved) society is willing to permit judgments that humane considerations warrant withholding life-sustaining medical interventions when life-threatening conditions arise. In theory, the suffering
and indignity of the individual may justify such determinations "in the
best interests" of the patient. The problem comes in implementing that
theory. For it is difficult to assess the level of suffering and sense of
degradation of persons who have reached such deteriorated states. The
appropriate fates of Claire Conroy, Joseph Saikewicz, Mary Hier, and
Joseph Storar were not easy to determine. At the extreme, in cases of

permanent coma or a permanent noncognitive state, some concensus is beginning to emerge that such a status is sufficiently degrading that omission of further medical intervention is tolerable. Beyond this class of patients, the legal steps will, understandably, be hesitant. At the very least, persons asked to shape the medical fates of the extremely debilitated, waning patient will be constantly made aware that the patient's interests rather than familial, medical, or societal expediency determine the ultimate decision. With those caveats in mind, there will still be some instances when humane concern will prompt decisions not to administer antibiotics or artificial resuscitation or even artificial nutrition to patients whose tortured existences could otherwise be protracted for extended periods. Procedural precautions, such as those discussed in chapter 5, are in order in such instances to ensure that the decisions are consistent with "quality of life" from the perspective of the patient rather than from some perspective of social worth. If this critical distinction is not maintained, then the proverbial slippery slope will really lie in front of the severely disabled population. If the distinction is maintained, then "death with dignity" may be taken from the realm of the slogan and made a part of the reality of life in America.

NOTES

Chapter I: Decisions By Competent Patients

1. 362 So.2d 160 (1978), aff'd 379 So.2d 359 (Fla. 1980).
2. Id. at 164.
3. In re *Quinlan*, 70 N.J. 10, 355 A.2d 647, 663 (1976).
4. In re *Colyer*, 99 Wash.2d 114, 660 P.2d 738, 742 (1983).
5. 362 So.2d at 162.
6. *Superintendent of Belchertown v. Saikewicz*, 370 N.E.2d 417, 426 (Mass. 1977).
7. See Matter of *Storar*, 52 N.Y.2d 363, 438 N.Y.S.2d 266, 420 N.E.2d 64, 70–71 (1981); *Randolph v. City of New York*, N.Y.L.J. (Sup. Ct. 10/12/84). See also In re *Conroy*, 486 A.2d 1209 (N.J. 1985).
8. See *Runyon v. McCrary*, 427 U.S. 160 (1976); *Village of Belle Terre v. Borass*, 416 U.S. 1 (1974). See generally *Roberts v. U.S. Jaycees*, 104 S.Ct. 3244, 3249–50 (1984).
9. *Griswold v. Connecticut*, 381 U.S. 479, 493 (1965) (Goldberg, J., concurring).
10. Matter of *Eichner*, 73 A.D.2d 431, 459 (N.Y. App. Div., 2d Dep't 1980).
11. California Health & Safety Code #7185 et seq.
12. Id. at #7186.
13. *Union Pacific Ry. v. Botsford*, 141 U.S. 250, 251 (1891).
14. *Natanson v. Kline*, 186 Kan. 393, 350 P.2d 1093, 1104 (1960).
15. President's Commission for the Study of Ethical Problems in Medicine and Biomedical and Behavioral Research, "Making Health Care Decisions" (Oct. 1982), p. 46. (hereinafter cited as "President's Commission").
16. See In re *Boyd*, 403 A.2d 744 (D.C. Ct. App. 1979); Brooks, "The Constitutional Right to Refuse Antipsychotic Medications," Bull. Amer. Acad. Psych. & Law 8:179 (1980).
17. *McKaskle v. Wiggins*, 104 S.Ct. 944, 950 (1984).
18. In re *Conroy*, 486 A.2d 1209 (N.J. 1985). For a commentary on *Conroy*, see Cantor, "*Conroy*, Best Interests, and the Handling of Dying Patients," 37 Rutgers L. Rev. 543 (1985).
19. See *Estate of Leach v. Shapiro*, 469 N.E.2d 1047 (Ohio App. 1984); *Randolph v. City of New York*, N.Y.L.J. (Sup. Ct. 1984).
20. See *Roberts v. United States Jaycees*, 104 S.Ct. 3244, 3250 (1984).
21. *Estate of Leach*, supra, note 19.
22. *Bartling v. Superior Court*, 163 Cal. App. 3d 186 (1984).
23. In re *Lydia E. Hall Hospital*, 116 Misc.2d 477, 455 N.Y.S.2d 706 (Sup.Ct. 1982).
24. Id. at 488. See also *New York Times*, 6/24/86, p. B1, reporting a New Jersey decision allowing a thirty-seven-year-old woman to reject a respirator which would have prolonged her existence for 6 to 12 months.
25. *Newark Star Ledger*, 2/3/84, p. 8.
26. In re *Conroy*, 486 A.2d 1209 (N.J. 1985).
27. See Brown & Thompson, "Nontreatment of Fever in Extended Care Facilities," 300 N. Eng. J. Med. 1246 (1979).
28. President's Commission for the Study of Ethical Problems in Medicine

and Biological and Behavioral Research, "Deciding to Forego Life-Sustaining Treatment" (1983), p. 97.

29. President's Commission, supra note 28, at 63.

30. *Randolph v. City of New York,* N.Y.L.J. (Sup. Ct. 1984).

31. Liacos, "Dilemmas of Dying," in Legal & Ethical Aspects of Treating Critically and Terminally Ill Patients (A. Doudera & J. Peters, eds. 1982), pp. 153–54.

32. *John F. Kennedy Hospital v. Heston,* 279 A.2d 670 (N.J. 1971).

33. In re *Quinlan,* 355 A.2d at 663.

34. *John F. Kennedy Memorial Hospital v. Heston,* 279 A.2d 670, 673 (N.J. 1970) (Chief Justice Weintraub).

35. *Foody v. Manchester Memorial Hospital,* 482 A.2d 713, 718–19 (Conn. Super. 1984).

36. In re *Conroy,* 486 A.2d at 1226.

37. 376 N.E.2d 1232 (Mass. App. 1978).

38. Matter of *Quackenbush,* 383 A.2d 785 (N.J. Super. Ct., Morris Cty 1978).

39. See *Commissioner of Correction v. Myers,* 399 N.E.2d 452 (Mass. 1979) (dictum); *Lydia E. Hall Hospital,* supra note 23. Cf. In re *Spring,* 405 N.E.2d 115 (Mass. 1980). See also *Newark Star Ledger,* 1/2/86, p. 38.

40. See also *State v. Northern,* 563 S.W.2d 197 (Tenn. Ct. App. 1978); In re *Raasch,* #455–996 (Prob. Div., Milwaukee County Ct. ¹/₂₅/72).

41. In re *Quinlan,* 70 N.J. 10, 355 A.2d 647, 664 (1976).

42. Newark Star Ledger, supra note 25. For discussion of the nature of the medical treatment which a patient may reject, and discussion of whether "artificial feeding" may be deemed medical treatment for these purposes, see Chapter 2 infra.

43. 205 N.E.2d 435 (Ill. 1965).

44. Id. at 442.

45. 294 A.2d 372 (D.C. Dist. Ct. 1972).

46. *Application of the President of Georgetown College,* 331 F.2d 1000 (D.C. Cir.), cert. denied 377 U.S. 978 (1964); *United States v. George,* 239 F. Supp. 752, 753 (D. Conn. 1965); *Powell v. Columbia Presbyterian Medical Center,* 267 N.Y.S.2d 450 (Sup. Ct. 1965).

47. See In the Matter of *Georgetown Hospital,* 331 F.2d 1000 (D.C. Cir.), cert. denied 377 U.S. 978 (1964).

48. See In re *Osborne,* 294 A.2d 372 (D.C. Ct. App. 1972); *Randolph v. City of New York,* N.Y.L.J. (Sup. Ct. 1984). Cf. *A.B. v. C.,* 477 N.Y.S.2d 281, 283 (Sup. Ct. 1984).

49. See *Application of the President of Georgetown College,* and other cases cited in note 45, supra.

50. Katz, The Silent World of Doctor and Patient (1984), pp. 157–63.

51. On this subject, see Annas & Densberger, "Competence to Refuse Medical Treatment: Autonomy versus Paternalism," 15 Toledo L. Rev. 561 (1984).

52. See Hastings Cent. Rep., 15:2 (April 1985), p. 3.

53. Id.

54. 284 Ga. 832, 286 S.E.2d 715 (1982).

55. 87 A.D.2d 66, 450 N.Y.S.2d 623 (App. Div. 1982).

56. 450 N.Y.S. 2d at 624–25.

57. See In re *Caulk,* 480 N.E.2d 93 (N.H. 1984); *White v. Narick,* 292 S.E.2d 54 (W.Va. 1982); *Commissioner v. Myers,* 399 N.E.2d 452 (Mass. 1979). Note, "Should a Hunger-Striking Prisoner Be Allowed to Die," 25 *Boston College Law Review* 423 (1984); Note, "Force Feeding Hunger-Striking Prisoners: A Framework for Analysis," 35 *University of Florida Law Review* 99 (1983).

58. *New York Times,* 4/9/84, p. A-14. See G. Annas, "When Suicide Prevention

Becomes Brutality: The Case of Elizabeth Bouvia,: Hastings Cent. Rep. 14:2 (April 1984), p. 20. Note, "Elizabeth Bouvia v. Riverside Hospital," 15 *Golden Gate Law Review* 407 (1985); Kane, "Keeping Elizabeth Bouvia Alive for the Public Good," 15:6 Hastings Cent. Rep. (Dec. 1985), p. 5. See also *New York Times*, 4/17/86, p. 1 detailing a later appellate ruling in favor of Ms. Bouvia.

Chapter II: Dispelling the Myths

1. 195 Cal. Rptr. 484, 490 (Dist.Ct.App. 1983).
2. In re *Conroy*, 486 A.2d 1209 (N.J. 1985).
3. 362 So.2d 160,163 (1978), aff'd 379 So.2d 359 (Fla. 1980).
4. Where a patient is incompetent and has left no instructions, the patient's best interests become the principle guide to appropriate medical handling. The best interests concept will be examined below, in chapter 3.
5. President's Commission, supra note 28, chapter 1.
6. In re *Conroy*, 486 A.2d at 1235.
7. Id.
8. Brown & Thompson, 300 N. Eng. J. Med. 1246, 1248 (May 31, 1979).
9. Van Scoy-Mosher, "An Oncologist's Case for No-Code Orders," in Legal and Ethical Aspects of Treating Critically and Terminally Ill Patients (Doudera & Peters, eds. 1982); N.Y. Times, 9/23/84, p. 6E; Note, "A Structural Analysis of the Physician-Patient Relationship in No-code Decisionmaking," 93 Yale L.J. 362 (1983); Rabkin, "Orders Not to Resuscitate," 293 N. Eng. J. Med. 364 (1976).
10. Matter of *Dinnerstein*, 380 N.E.2d 134 (Mass. App. 1978); See also *Custody of a Minor*, 434 N.E.2d 601 (Mass. 1982); *New York Times*, 4/20/86, p. 36.
11. *Barber v. Superior Court*, 147 Cal. App.3d 1006, 195 Cal. Rptr. 484, 491 (Dist. Ct. App. 1983).
12. Callahan, "On Feeding the Dying," Hastings Cent. Rep. 13:5 (Oct. 1983), p. 22.
13. Steinbock, "The Removal of Mr. Herbert's Feeding Tube," Hastings Cent. Rep. (Oct. 1983), p.14.
14. See comments by Prof. Virginia Keeney of the U. of Louisville School of Medicine at 23 J. Fam. L. 212 (1984).
15. President's Commission, supra note 28, chapter 1.
16. Wanzer, Adelstein, Cranford, Federman, Hook, Moertel, Safar, Stone, Taussig, & Van Eys, "The Physician's Responsibility Toward Hopelessly Ill Patients," N.E. J. Med. 310:15 (April 12, 1984), at p.958.
17. Congress and a few state legislatures have sought to circumscribe the withholding of nutrition from defective newborns. Even then, the legislative prohibition usually allows for withholding of nutrition in "appropriate" cases. The medical handling of newborns is discussed in chapter 6, infra.
18. *Newark Star Ledger*, supra note 25.
19. *Zant v. Prevatte*, 286 S.E.2d 715 (Ga. 1982).
20. 147 Cal. App.3d 1006, 195 Ca. Rptr. 484 (Dist. Ct. App. 1983).
21. *Barber*, 147 Cal. App. 3d at 1017–1018.
22. In re *Conroy*, 486 A.2d 1209 (N.J. 1985).
23. In re *Conroy*, 486 A.2d at 1236. See also matter of *Jobes*, #C-4971-8SE (Ch. Div., Morris City, N.J. 4/23/86).
24. Id. But see *Brophy v. New England Sinai Hospital*, #85E0009-G1 (Mass. Prob. Ct. 10/21/85).
25. See In re *Hier*, 464 N.E.2d 959 (Mass. App. 1984).
26. This normally means that there must be a naturally occurring life-

threatening condition—as opposed to a self-induced fatal condition—facing the patient. As to self-induced conditions, see this chapter.

27. *A.B. v. C.*, 477 N.Y.S.2d 281 (Sup. Ct. 1984).

28. 362 So.2d 160, 162 (1978), aff'd 379 So.2d 359 (Fla. 1980).

29. Sacred Congregation for the Doctrine of the Faith, "Declaration on Euthanasia," (6/26/80), quoted in *New York Times*, 9/23/84, p. 6E.

30. See *Lydia E. Hall Hospital*, 116 Misc.2d 477, 455 N.Y.S.2d 706, 712 (Sup.Ct. 1982).

31. *Quinlan*, 355 A.2d at 665. For a similar and more recent expression differentiating suicide from rejection of life-preserving medical treatment, see In re *Conroy*, 486 A.2d 1209.

32. *John F. Kennedy Hospital v. Heston*, 58 N.J. 576, 279 A.2d 670 (1971) (overruled in part in In re *Conroy*, supra); In re *Georgetown College*, 331 F.2d 1000 (D.C. Cir.) cert. denied 377 U.S. 978 (1964). See also *United States v. George*, 239 F. Supp. 752 (D. Conn. 1965); *Collins v. Davis*, 254 N.Y.S.2d 666 (Sup. Ct. 1964); *Powell v. Columbia Presbyterian Hospital*, 267 N.Y.S.2d 450 (Sup. Ct. 1965). See generally Sherlock, "For Everything There is a Season: The Right to Die in the U.S.," 1982 Brigham Young L. Rev. 545 (1982); Chapman, "Fateful Treatment Choices for Critically Ill Adults," 37 Ark. L. Rev. 908 (1984).

33. In re *Georgetown College*, 331 F.2d at 1008–09.

34. Sherlock, supra note 32, 1982 Brigham Young L. Rev. at 557.

35. *New York Times*, April 9, 1984, p. A-14, col. 6; Annas, "The Case of Elizabeth Bouvia," supra note 58 chapter 1.

36. Williams, *The Sanctity of Life and the Criminal Law* (Faber & Faber Publishers, London: 1956), p. 292.

37. See, e.g., E. Diamond, "Treatment versus Nontreatment for the Handicapped Newborn," in Infanticide and the Handicapped Newborn (D. Horan & M. Delahoyde, eds. 1982), p. 55; J. Robertson, "Organ Donations by Incompetents and the Substituted Judgment Doctrine," 76 Colum. L. Rev. 48, 49–51 (1976); H. Hyde, "The Human Life Bill: Some Issues and Answers," 27 N.Y.U. L. Rev. 1077 (1982).

38. *Newark Star Ledger*, Feb. 16, 1984, p. 47, col. 1.

39. Malcolm, "To Suffer a Prolonged Illness or Elect to Die," *New York Times*, 12/16/84, p. 1, col. 5. See also *New York Times*, 3/28/86, p. B2, concerning rejection of dialysis.

40. *New York Times*, 11/17/84, p. 9. *Bartling v. Superior Court*, 163 Cal. App.3d 186 (1984).

41. The recent President's Commission for the Study of Ethical Problems in Medicine recognized that "quality of life" was a term subject to varying definitions. The Commission therefore emphasized that quality and value of life must be assessed from the patient's perspective without regard to outside persons' views of the patient's social value or utility. See President's Commission, "Deciding to Forego Life-Sustaining Treatment," supra note 28, chapter 1. See also In re *Conroy*, 486 A.2d at 1232–33, expressing aversion to considerations of "personal worth or social utility of another's life, or the value of that life to others" in the calculus of when to withdraw life-preserving treatment from an incompetent dying person.

Chapter III. Handling Incompetent Patients: Decision-Making Criteria

1. 70 N.J. 10, 355 A.2d 647 (1976). For more detailed commentary on *Quinlan*, see Cantor, "*Quinlan*, Privacy, and the Handling of Incompetent Dying Patients," 30 Rutgers L. Rev. 243 (1977).

2. As noted above, this issue of who can make a terminal decision for an incompetent patient will be examined in greater detail in chapter 5.

3. 355 A.2d at 671.

4. Id. at 653.

5. Id at 667–68.

6. As of March 1985, Karen Ann Quinlan had survived not only removal of the respirator, but cessation of antibiotics. She lay comatose, curled in a fetal position, weighing between sixty and seventy pounds. Nurses were turning her periodically, attending to bed sores, and responding to arm and leg spasms. Nourishment through a naso-gastric tube was being continued. See Ragonese, "Quinlans Reflect on Decade of Agony and Love," *Newark Star Ledger,* 3/17/85, p. 1. Ms. Quinlan expired on June 12, 1985.

7. 486 A.2d 1209 (N.J. 1985).

8. 457 A.2d 1232 (N.J. Super. Ct., Ch. Div. 1983).

9. In re *Conroy,* 464 A,.2d 303 (N.J. App. Div. 1983).

10. 486 A.2d at 1231.

11. See *In re Hamlin,* 689 P.2d 1372 (Wash. 1984).

12. Matter of *Spring,* 405 N.E.2d 115, 119, 121 (Mass. 1980).

13. *Conroy,* 486 A.2d at 1229.

14. *Conroy,* 486 A.2d at 1230. See also *John F. Kennedy Hospital v. Bludworth,* 432 So.2d 611, 620 (Fla. 4th App. Dist. 1983). "Consistency" as used in *Conroy* with regard to a patient's prior expressions, probably has two aspects. First, the patient's statements should be internally consistent, offering some clear guidance to decision-makers. Second, if there is some change in a patient's expressed attitude, the more recent instruction, if clearcut, must presumably be heeded.

15. Helfiker, "Allowing the Debilitated to Die," N.E. J. Med., 3/24/83, at p.718. See also Van Scoy-Mosher, "An Oncologist's Case for No-Code Orders," in Legal & Ethical Aspects of Treating Critically & Terminally Ill Patients (Doudera & Peters, eds. 1982), p.17.

16. President's Commission for the Study of Ethical Problems in Medicine and Biomedical and Behavioral Research, "Making Health Care Decisions" (1982), pp.49–50. As one authority in the field has commented: "It is an assault on human dignity to impose treatment on adults despite wishes they clearly and knowledgeably expressed while coherent and competent." Veatch, Death, Dying and the Biological Revolution (1976), at 163.

17. See matter of *Eichner,* 73 A.D.2d 431, 426 N.Y.S.2d 507 (2d Dept 1980), aff'd in relevant part in Matter of *Storar,* 52 N.Y.2d 363, 438 N.Y.S.2d 266, 420 N.E.2d 64 (1981); In re *Severns,* 425 A.2d 156, 158 (Del. Ch. Div. 1980). See also *John F. Kennedy Hospital v. Bludworth,* 432 So.2d 611, for an example of fulfillment of a "living will" stating the patient's preferences with regard to terminal care.

18. See Walton, Ethics of Withdrawal of Life Support Systems (1983), p. 114; Veatch, "An Ethical Framework for Terminal Care Decisions," J. Am. Geriatrics Socy 32:9 (1984), p. 666; Robertson, "Organ Donations by Incompetents and the Substituted Judgment Doctrine," 76 Colum. L. Rev. 48, 65 (1976).

19. 660 P.2d 738, 748 (1983).

20. 357 N.W.2d 332 (Minn. 1984).

21. 405 N.E.2d 115, 123 (Mass. 1980).

22. The *Conroy* decision is partially responsive to these complaints. That court acknowledged that in many instances a guardian cannot be "clearly satisfied" as to what the incompetent patient's subjective preference would be. Moreover, the Court indicated that "self-determination" as a touchstone of decision-making must then be melded with "best interests" analysis, as the Court tried to do in its "limited-objective" test of the best interests of an incompetent patient. See also *Foody v. Manchester Memorial Hospital,* 482 A.2d 713, 721 (Conn. Super. 1984).

23. President's Commission, "Deciding to Forego Life-Sustaining Treatment," supra note 28 in chapter 1; President's Commission, "Making Health Care Decisions", supra note 16. For a contrary view, see Katz, "Limping Is No Sin: Reflections on 'Making Health Care Decisions' " 6 Cardozo L. Rev. 243, 261–64 (1984).

24. *Conroy,* 486 A.2d at 1231.

25. Id. at 1232.

26. "Net" pain and suffering is defined as the pain which will be suffered if treatment is continued, discounted by the pain which will be suffered during the dying process if the treatment is withdrawn. Ibid.

27. Id. at 1232.

28. Id.

29. President's Commission, supra note 28, in chapter 1. President's Commission, "Making Health Care Decisions," supra note 16.

30. See Matter of *Torres,* 357 N.W.2d 332, 337 (Minn. 1984); *State Department of Human Services v. Northern,* 563 S.W.2d 197, 214–15 (Tenn. Ct. App. 1978); *Matter of Eichner,* 73 A.D.2d 431, 451 (2d Dept. 180), modified In re *Storar,* 52 N.Y.2d 363, 538 N.Y.S.2d 266, 420 N.E.2d 64 (1981); *Foody v. Manchester Memorial Hospital,* 482 A.2d 713, 721 (Conn. Super. 1984). Cf. In re *Grady,* 85 N.J. 235, 426, 467, 471, 475 (1981).

31. *Conroy,* 486 A.2d at 1232 (emphasis added).

32. Id. at 1231.

33. Id. at 1232.

34. Id. at 1233.

35. A poignant reminder of the frustration and suffering of some helpless, deteriorating patients was provided in the recent *Bartling* case in California. There, a competent patient suffering from several potentially terminal conditions, including emphysema and cancer, was maintained on a respirator contrary to his express wishes. His written pleas for relief cited his "unbearable, degrading, and dehumanizing" existence, as well as "the humiliating indignity" of having every bodily need and function tended by others. *Bartling v. Superior Court,* 163 Cal. App.3d 186, 188 (Calif. Dist. Ct. App. 1984).

36. Such emotional feelings as frustration, embarrassment, and humiliation may well be connected to the patient's deteriorated physical and/or intellectual state, i.e., to a personally distasteful quality of existence. The President's Commission noted level of functioning and quality of existence as relevant factors in decision-making for the incompetent. President's Commission, "Deciding to Forego Life-Sustaining Treatment" supra note 28, chap. 1. I suggest that such factors are deemed relevant because they relate both to emotional suffering of an incompetent patient, and to widely shared perceptions of human dignity and humane treatment. The implication is that there is a level of functioning and quality of life at which continued maintenance is inhumane, or a violation of human dignity. See chapter 1, infra for further discussion of this point.

37. See, e.g., President's Commission, "Deciding to Forego Life-Sustaining Treatment," supra note at 134–35; Gaylin, "Who Speaks for the Child?" in Who Speaks for the Child (Gaylin & Macklin, eds. 1982), p. 6; *Barber v. Superior Court,* 195 Calif. Rptr. 484, 493 (Dist. Ct. App. 1983). The President's Commission even accepts burdens on surrounding loved ones as a legitimate factor in assessing the best interests of the incompetent patient. See President's Commission, supra note 16, at 135–36.

38. In re *Conroy,* 486 A.2d at 1217. Despite the uncertainty of the testimony about Mrs. Conroy's capacity to experience pain, the trial court had concluded that death by starvation—upon removal of the naso-gastric tube—would be painful for her. See 457 A.2d at 1236. This conclusion, implying an inability to provide analgesic relief during starvation, seems suspect. See *Barber v. Superior*

Court, 195 Cal. Rptr. 484 (Dist. Ct. App. 1983); In the Matter of *Mary Hier,* 18 Mass. App. 200, 464 N.E.2d 959 (Mass. App. 1984).

39. *Conroy,* 486 A.2d at 1217. For another recent example of the difficulty of assessing the feelings of semi-comatose patients, see matter of *Jobes,* #C-4971-85E (Ch. Div., Morris County N.J., 4/23/86).

40. The New Jersey Supreme Court acknowledged the uncertainty of assessing benefits and burdens for non-communicative, virtually insensate individuals:

> Often it is unclear whether and to what extent a patient such as Claire Conroy is capable of, or is in fact, experiencing pain. Similarly, medical experts are often unable to determine with any degree of certainty the extent of a nonverbal person's intellectual function or the depth of his emotional life. 486 A.2d at 1233.

41. Donovan, "Cancer Pain: You Can Help!", Nursing Clinics of North America 17:4 (Dec. 1982), at 713–14.

42. *Conroy,* 486 A.2d at 1243.

43. *Leach v. Akron General Medical Center,* 68 Ohio Misc. 1, 426 N.E.2d 809 (Comm. Pl. 1980); *Foody v. Manchester Memorial Hospital,* 482 A.2d 713 (Conn. Super. 1984). Cf. Matter of *Dinnerstein,* 380 N.E.2d 134 (Mass. App. 1978).

44. *Griswold v. Connecticut,* 381 U.S. 479, 493 (Goldberg, J. concurring).

45. 70 N.J. 10, 355 A.2d 647 (1976).

46. While *Quinlan* spoke only to removal of a respirator, *Conroy* spoke to termination of artificial nourishment as well.

47. The *Quinlan* court asserted that its determination to authorize cessation of life-preserving treatment "should be accepted by a society the overwhelming majority of whose members would . . . exercise such a choice in the same way for themselves.

48. *Conroy,* 486 A.2d at 1247 (Handler, J., dissenting)

49. Id. at 1250.

50. Id. at 1246.

51. President's Commission, "Making Health Care Decisions," supra note 16.

52. See AMA Jud. Council Op. 2.11 (1/10/81); Wanzer, Adelstein, et al "The Physician's Responsibility toward Hopelessly Ill Patients," N.Eng. J. Med. 310:15 (4/12/84), p. 958.

53. In re *Torres,* 357 N.W.2d 332, 337 (Minn. 1984); *John F. Kennedy Hospital v. Bludworth,* 452 So.2d 921 (Fla. 1984); In re *Colyer,* 99 Wash.2d 114, 660 P.2d 738 (1983); Matter of *Storar,* 52 N.Y.2d 363, 438 N.Y.S.2d 266, 420 N.E.2d 64 (1981); *Severns v. Wilmington Medical Center,* 421 A.2d 1334 (1980).

54. Wanzer, supra note 16, chapter 2. See also Statement of the Council on Ethical and Judicial Affairs of the AMA, 3/15/86, cited in *New York Times,* 3/17/86, p. 5.

55. See cases cited in note 43, supra.

56. In *Foody,* 482 A.2d at 717, the semicomatose patient was classified as "awake, but unaware." The patient could swallow and could respond in primitive fashion to some stimuli such as noise. In *Brophy v. New England Sinai Hospital,* #85E0009-G1 (Mass. Prob. Ct. 10/21/85), the patient was also classified as "awake, but unaware." The court authorized a treatment approach under which most life-preserving medical care could be omitted, but the court refused to authorize cessation of artificial nourishment. This case is discussed in chapter 4. See also Matter of *Jobes,* supra note 39.

57. 457 A.2d 1232, 1236 (N.J. Super. Ct. Ch. Div. 1983).

58. See Wanzer, supra note 16, chapter 2; Walton, *Ethics of Withdrawal of Life-Support Systems* (1983), pp. 210, 218.

59. This analysis of human dignity is confined to the previously competent individual. Such a person has had the opportunity to form and express prefer-

ences about acceptable lifestyles or levels of disability, and how the dying process should be shaped. It is also possible to make certain assumptions about such a person's likely emotional needs and feelings based on prior expressions and patterns of conduct.

It is much harder to assess the needs, feelings, and preferences of persons who have always been severely retarded or deranged. See Chapman, "Fateful Treatment Choices for Critically Ill Adults, Part I: The Judicial Model," 37 Ark. L. Rev. 908, 936 (1984); Walton, Ethics of Withdrawal of Life-Support Systems (1983), pp. 47, 55. To be sure, such persons are fully entitled to be treated with human dignity. The problem is assessing the significance of factors such as dependence, helplessness, or embarrassment for such persons. In other words, extent of emotional suffering or tolerable level of debilitation will not be the same for such persons as for formerly competent and vigorous individuals. My discussion at this point is limited to the latter class of patients.

60. Because the record was scanty about the use of physical restraint on Mrs. Conroy, the New Jersey Supreme Court indicated that the matter should be investigated and considered by any subsequent decision-maker in a comparable case. 486 A.2d at 1243–44.

61. See Matter of *Eichner,* 73 A.D. 2d 431 (2d Dept. 1980), modified in Matter of *Storar,* 52 N.Y.2d 363, 438 N.Y.S.2d 266, 420 N.E.2d 64 (1981); In re *Mary Hier,* 18 Mass. App. 200, 464 N.E.2d 959, 946–66 (Mass. App. 1984). In *Mary Hier,* the court went so far as to regard the deranged ninety-two-year-old patient's resistance to feeding tubes as "a plea for privacy and personal dignity." 464 N.E.2d at 965. Without some finding that the patient understood the fatal consequences of her resistance, it seems presumptuous to regard her action as a considered request for termination of treatment. However, the court was on firmer ground in treating Mrs. Hier's conduct as at least indicative of a burden being felt during the continued life-preserving medical intervention. 464 N.E.2d at 966.

62. See In re *Caulk,* 480 A.2d 93, 99 (N.H. 1984) (dissent in case ordering forced feeding of a hunger-striking prisoner).

Chapter IV: Trouble Spots on the Horizon

1. *New York Times,* 12/23/84, p. 1.
2. *New York Times,* 9/23/84, p. 6E.
3. *Newark Star Ledger,* June 16, 1985, Section 1, p.41.
4. E.g., *Conroy,* 486 A.2d at 1233; *John F. Kennedy Hospital v. Bludworth,* 452 So.2d 921, 926 (Fla. 1984). A notable exception to the trend is Matter of *Storar,* 52 N.Y.2d 363, 438 N.Y.S.2d 266, 420 N.E.2d 64 (1981), where New York State's highest court overturned a very plausible terminal decision (to cease blood transfusions to an incompetent, dying cancer patient suffering painful and disturbing side effects from the transfusions) even though the patient's devoted mother felt that the decision was in the patient's best interests. See generally Veatch, "Limits of Guardian Treatment Refusal: A Reasonableness Standard," Am. J.L. & Med. 427 (1984).
5. See Walton, Ethics of Withdrawal of Life-Support Systems (1983), pp. 80, 96; Beresford, Book Review, 57 N.Y.U. L. Rev. 1273, 1276–77 (1982).
6. Hyde, "The Human Life Bill: Some Issues and Answers," 27 N.Y.U. L. Rev. 1077 (1982); Gelfand, "Euthanasia and the Terminally Ill Patient," 63 Neb. L. Rev. 741 (1984).
7. Kleiman, "Uncertainty Clouds Care of the Dying," N.Y. Times, 1/18/85, p. B1, quoting Dr. John Rowe of Harvard Medical School.

8. For a broad analysis of the legal and economic policy implications of providing expensive lifesaving treatment, see Mehlman, "Rationing Expensive Lifesaving Medical Treatments," 1985 Wis. L. Rev. 239 (1985).

9. President's Commission, "Deciding to Forego Life-Sustaining Treatment," supra note 28, chapter 1.

10. In mid-1985, news reports described how hospitals in New Jersey vigorously seek alternative facilities—including home care and hospices—for comatose patients who have been removed from life-support machinery but whose medical condition has stabilized. *Newark Star Ledger,* June 16, 1985, Section 1, p. 41.

11. See Cassell, "Deciding to Forego Life-Sustaining Treatment: Implications for Policy in 1985," 6 Cardozo L. Rev. 287, 288–95 (1984).

12. See *Superintendent of Belchertown v. Saikewicz,* 370 N.E.2d 417, 431 (Mass. 1977).

13. President's Commission, "Deciding to Forego Life-Sustaining Treatment," supra note 28, chapter 1.

14. In re *Torres,* 357 N.W.2d 332, 339 (Minn. 1984); *John F. Kennedy Hospital v. Bludworth,* 432 So.2d 611, 618 (Fla. 4th App. Dist. 1983).

15. See *Conroy,* 486 A.2d at 1232–33; *Saikewicz,* 370 N.E.2d at 432. Cf. Burt, "The Ideal of Community in the Work of the President's Commission," 6 Cardozo L. Rev. 267, 279–81 (1984) (concerning altruism and withholding of treatment from severely handicapped newborns).

16. Wanzer, Adelstein & others, "The Physician's Response Toward Hopelessly Ill Patients," 310:15 N.Eng. J. Med. (4/12/84), p. 957.

17. Opinions of the Judicial Council, AMA (1982), pp. 9–10.

18. In a recent case concerning whether to reimplant a feeding tube in a highly debilitated ninety-two-year-old incompetent woman, one physician opposed further medical intervention because of the resources already expended in maintaining the patient's marginal existence (contrary to her ostensible will). The doctor reportedly testified that it would be "economically untenable" to proceed with reinsertion of the tube. Annas, "The Case of Mary Hier: When Substituted Judgment Becomes Sleight of Hand, Hastings Cent. Rep. 14:4 (Aug. 1984), p.23.

19. Kleiman, "Changing Way of Death: Some Agonizing Choices," *New York Times,* 1/14/85, p.1.

20. See Mehlman, supra note 8.

21. Sacred Congregation for the Doctrine of the Faithful, "Declaration on Euthanasia" (1980), reprinted in President's Commission, "Deciding to Forego Life-Sustaining Treatment," supra note 28, chapter 1.

22. See chapter 4.

23. See Brown & Thompson, "Nontreatment of Fever in Extended Care Facilities," 300 N.Eng. J. Med. 1246, 1247–49 (May 31, 1979).

24. *Superintendent of Belchertown v. Saikewicz,* 370 N.E.2d 417 (Mass. 1977).

25. Id. at 422.

26. 370 N.E.2d at 428.

27. E.g., Besdine, "Decisions to Withhold Treatment from Nursing Home Residents," J. Am. Geriat. Socy 31:10 (1984), p. 602; Helfiker, "Allowing the Debilitated to Die," 308 N.Eng. J. Med. 716 (1983); Brown, "Non-treatment of Fever in Extended Care Facilities," 300 N.Eng. J. Med. 1246 (1979).

28. See *Barber v. Superior Court,* 195 Cal. Rptr. 484 (Dist. Ct. App. 1983); In re *Severns,* 425 A.2d 156, 160 (Del. Ch. 1980); Hastings Center Report (Aug. 1986), p. 40.

But see *New York Times,* 10/23/85, p. A-16, reporting the refusal of a Massachusetts judge to authorize removal of a feeding tube from a permanently vegetative patient. This case, known as *Brophy,* is discussed in chapter 4. See also matter of *Jobes,* infra note 32.

29. Wanzer, Adelstein, & others, supra note 16. See also statements of the AMA Council on Ethical and Judicial Affairs, quoted in *New York Times,* 3/17/86, p. 5.

30. In the Matter of *Mary Hier,* 18 Mass. App. 200, 464 N.E.2d 959 (Mass. App. 1984). There, the court originally approved withholding of the surgery, but later received additional medical testimony which prompted a reversal of the original decision.

31. The issue of artificial feeding is discussed in greater length in chapter 2, at pp. 14–26.

32. As of September 1986, this very issue was being litigated in New Jersey. There, a guardian of a permanently comatose patient was seeking to remove artificial nourishment even though the patient would survive for more than a year if feeding were maintained. See *New York Times,* 11/5/85, p. B3. In April 1986, a lower court judge in New Jersey rules that the artificial feeding could be discontinued. Matter of *Jobes,* #C-4971-85 E (Ch. Div., Morris County N.J. 4/23/86).

In Massachusetts, in October 1985, a judge refused to authorize a removal of a feeding tube from a forty-eight-year-old who had suffered permanent brain damage from a broken blood vessel in the brain. The medical projection was that the immobile, incontinent, and vegetative patient could live for many years if feeding were maintained. The judge was willing to authorize withholding of "special measures," but not to discontinue nutrition. *New York Times,* 10/23/85, p. A-16. This case *(Brophy)* is discussed below.

33. *Brophy v. New England Sinai Hospital,* #85E0009-G1 (Mass. Prob. Ct. 10/21/85).

34. Id., slip opinion at 42.

35. Id. at 43.

36. Id. at 20. In April 1985, during an attack of bronchitis, antibiotics were intravenously administered to Mr. Brophy. Because of damage to the veins at that time doctors projected that any future antibiotics treatment would have to be administered through the subclavian vein in the chest.

37. Id. at 28–29.

38. Id. at 30–32. See also Statement of the AMA Council on Ethical and Judicial Affairs, *New York Times,* 3/17/86, p. 5.

39. Ironically, in April 1985, while the matter was pending before the court, antibiotics were administered after a bronchitis attack and the patient was saved from a potentially fatal infection and maintained in his present indefinite limbo.

40. Matter of *Dinnerstein,* 380 N.E.2d 134 (Mass. App. 1978). See Note, "A Structural Analysis of the Physician-Patient Relationship in No-Code Decision-making," 93 Yale L.J. 362 (1983).

41. See, e.g., Note, "No-Code Orders versus Resuscitation: The Decision to Withhold Life-Prolonging Treatment for the Terminally Ill," 26 Wayne L. Rev. 139 (1979); Van Scoy-Mosher, "An Oncologist's Case for No-Code Orders," in Legal & Ethical Aspects of Treating Critically & Terminally Ill Patients (Doudera & Peters eds. 1982), p. 14; *New York Times,* 9/23/84, p. 6E.

42. See Note, "No-Code Orders," supra note 41 at 141; Nat'l Conf. on Standards for Cardiopulmonary Resuscitation, 227 J.A.M.A. 837, 838 (1974).

Chapter V: Who Decides for the Incompetent?

1. In the Matter of *Quinlan,* 70 N.J. 10, 355 A.2d 647 (1976).
2. *Saickewicz,* supra note 120, 370 N.E.2d at 435.

3. For discussion of the proper allocation of decision-making authority on behalf of incompetent adults, see, e.g., Baron, "Medical Paternalism and the Rule of Law: A Reply to Dr. Relman," 4 Am. J. L. & Med. 337 (1979); J. Childress, Who Should Decide? (1982), pp. 172–75.

4. Matter of *Colyer*, 99 Wash.2d 114, 660 P.2d 738 (1983).

5. *Colyer*, was modified in 1984 in In re *Hamlin*, 689 P.2d 1372, 1376–1377 (Wash. 1984). The court decided not to require a formal guardianship proceeding where family members are present to make decisions in conjunction with treating physicians and a prognosis committee.

6. President's Commission, "Deciding to Forego Life-Sustaining Treatment," supra note 16, chapter 3.

7. Id. at 128.

8. *Quinlan*, supra note 1, 355 A.2d at 669.

9. President's Commission, "Deciding to Forego Life-Sustaining Treatment," supra note 16, chapter 3. For other discussions of institutional ethics committees, see R. Cranford and A. Doudera, Institutional Ethics Committees and Health Care Decision-Making (1984). The idea of an institutional ethics committee has great currency in the context of decision-making for defective newborns. That topic will be examined in chapter 6.

10. See generally Randal, "Are Ethics Committees Alive and Well?" 13:6 Hastings Cent. Rep. (Dec. 1983), p. 10; Levine, "Questions and Answers about Ethics Committees," Hastings Cent. Rep., Aug. 1984, at 9.

11. See *Newark Star Ledger*, March 1, 1984, pp. 1, 6. Many of New Jersey's hospitals utilize "prognosis" committees—bodies consisting of medical personnel whose function is primarily to review the medical status of the patient whose treatment may be terminated. See *Newark Star Ledger*, June 16, 1985, Section 1, p. 41.

12. For commentary on *Saikewicz*, and for arguments supporting judicial involvement in decision-making, see Baron, "Assuring 'Detached but Passionate Investigation and Decision': The Role of Guardian ad Litem in *Saikewicz*-type Cases," 4 Am. J. L. & Med. 111 (1978); Baron, supra note 3.

13. Note, "Appointing an Agent to Make Medical Treatment Choices," 84 Colum. L. Rev. 985, 995 (1984).

14. See the list contained in Chapman, "Fateful Treatment Choices for Critically Ill Adults, Part I: The Judicial Model," 37 Ark. L. Rev. 908, 960 (1984). To that list of patients who died awaiting the outcome of litigation aimed at securing a merciful death add Mr. Bartley in California and Mrs. Conroy in New Jersey.

15. In re *Torres*, 357 N.W.2d 332, 341 (Minn. 1984). While the court in *Torres* found that a judicial order was appropriate in the particular case before it, it indicated that normally consultation between physician and family, with approval of an ethics committee, would suffice for decision-making on behalf of an incompetent, dying patient.

16. Matter of *Colyer*, 99 Wash.2d 114, 660 P.2d 738 (1983).

17. See *Severns v. Wilmington Medical Center*, 421 A.2d 1334 (Del. 1980); *Leach v. Akron General Medical Center*, 68 Ohio Misc. 1, 426 N.E.2d 809 (C.Pl. 1980); see also *Estate of Leach v. Shapiro*, 469 N.E.2d 1097 (Ohio App. 1984).

18. See Ark. Stat. Ann §§82—3801 to 03 (Supp. 1983); N.C. Gen. Stat. §90—322 (Supp. 1983); Va. Code §§54—325.8:1 to :12 (Supp. 1984); Fla. Stat. §§765.01 to .07 (West Supp. 1985); Or. Rev. Stat. §97.050–.090 (amended 1983 Or. Laws c. 526 §3; N.W. Stat. Ann. §§27-7-4, 27-7-8.1 (1984 Supp.). See generally note, "Proxy Decision-Making for the Terminally Ill: The Virginia Approach," 70 Va. L. Rev. 1269, 1275 (1984).

19. Va. Code §54-325.8:2 (Supp. 1985).

20. N.C. Gen. Stat. §90-322; Or. Rev. Stat. §97.050-.090 (amended 1983 Or. Laws c.526 §3.)

21. President's Commission, Making Health Care Decisions (1981), p. 185.

22. Chapman, supra note 14, 37 Ark. L. Rev. at 970.

23. See, e.g., Note, "Appointing an Agent," supra note 13, 84 Colum. L. Rev. at 995; Note, "Proxy Decision-Making," supra note 18, 70 Va. L. Rev.

24. Liacos, "Dilemmas of Dying," in Legal and Ethical Aspects of Treating Critically and Terminally Ill Patients (Doudera & Peters eds. 1982), p. 155.

25. 405 N.E.2d 115 (Mass. 1980).

26. Id. at 121.

27. In re *Torres*, 357 N.W.2d 332, 341 n.4 (1984).

28. In re *Hamlin*, 689 P.2d at 1377.

29. *Barber v. Superior Court*, 195 Cal. Rptr. 484, 492–93 (Dist. Ct. App. 1983); *Severns v. Wilmington Medical Center*, 421 A.2d 1334, 1338 (Del. 1980); *John F. Kennedy Hospital v. Bludworth*, 452 So.2d 921 (Fla. 1984).

30. 452 So.2d 921 (Fla. 1984).

31. Id. at 926. The court indicated that this process should be applied in *Bludworth* and "similar cases." The intendment of "similar cases" was not clear. It could refer to permanently comatose patients, or it could refer to patients who have left written instructions for their medical handling, as was the case there. For another case allowing a guardian and physician to make a termination decision for a patient who had left clear instructions, see Matter of *Eichner*, 73 A.D.2d 431 (2d Dept. 1980), aff'd in Matter of *Storar* 438 N.Y.S.2d 266, 420 N.E.2d 64, 74 (N.Y. 1981).

32. See, e.g., Wanzer et al. "The Physician's Responsibility toward Hopelessly Ill Patients," 310 N. Eng. J. Med. 955, 958 (1984).

33. See sources cited in note 18, supra.

34. See generally Brooks, "The Constitutional Right to Refuse Antipsychotic Medication," 8:179 Bull. Amer. Acad. Psych. & Law (1980).

35. For a view criticizing the procedures outlined in *Conroy* as overly rigorous, see Annas, "When Procedures Limit Rights: From *Quinlan* to *Conroy*," Hastings Cent. Rep., 15:2 (April 1985), pp. 25–26.

36. See Besdine, "Decisions to Withhold Treatment from Nursing Home Residents, 31:10 J. Am. Ger. Socy (1984) at p. 605 for a suggestion that nursing homes might use an "ethics issues team" to guide an attending physician in the absence of a reliable next of kin, or in the event that close family disagree about a particular decision.

37. Letter to the Editor, *New York Times*, 10/3/84, p. A-26.

38. See note, "Appointing an Agent," supra note 13, 84 Colum. L. Rev. 1006–07.

39. For a comprehensive analysis of the durable power of attorney, see note, "Appointing an Agent," supra note 13. See also Uniform Durable Power of Attorney Act, 8 U.L.A. 511–18 (1983).

40. *Conroy*, 486 A.2d at 1230.

Chapter VI: Defective Infants

1. For descriptions of an array of neonatal anomalies see, e.g., R. Weir, Selective Nontreatment of Handicapped Newborns 38–49 (1984); Smith, "Life and Death Decisions in the Nursery: Standards and Procedures for Withholding Lifesaving Treatment from Infants," 27 N.Y.L. Sch. L. Rev. 1125 (1982).

2. See Strong, "The Tiniest Newborns," Hastings Cent. Rep., Feb. 1983, at 14–19; Meyer, "Protecting the Best Interests of the Child: Is the State the Necessary Blunt Instrument?," 1984 Ariz. St. L.J., 627, 629.

3. See, e.g., Gallo, "Spina Bifida: The State of the Art of Medical Management," Hastings Cent. Rep., Feb. 1984, at 10–13; Brown & McLone, "Treatment

Choices for the Infant with Meningomyelocele," in Infanticide and the Handicapped Newborn 69–75 (D. Horan & M. Delahoyde, eds. 1982).

4. Smith and Smith, "Selection for Treatment in Spina Bifida Cystica," 4 Brit. Med. J. 187, 196 (1973).

5. See Shatten and Chabon, "Decision-Making and the Right to Refuse Lifesaving Treatment for Defective Newborns," 3 J. Legal Med. 59, 65 n.30 (1982).

6. *Application of Cicero*, 101 Misc. 2d 669, 702 (N.Y. Sup. Ct. 1979).

7. *Maine Medical Center v. Houle*, No. 74-145 (Super. Ct. Cumberland County, Me., Feb. 14, 1974), noted in Note, "Birth-Defective Infants; A Standard for Nontreatment Decisions," 30 Stan. L. Rev. 599, 601 n.13 (1978).

8. See In re *Daniels*, No. 81-15577FJ101 (Cir. Ct. Dade County, Fla. June 23, 1981), noted in Portela, "The Elin Daniels Case: An Examination of the Legal, Medical, and Ethical Considerations Posed when Parents and Doctors Disagree on Whether to Treat a Defective Newborn," 18 The Forum 709 (1983).

9. See In re *Obernauer*, (Juv. & Dom. Rel. Ct. Morris County, N.J. Dec. 22, 1970), noted in Note, "Birth-Defective Infants," supra note 7; *Newark Star Ledger*, Oct. 3, 1973, at 32, col. 8 (reporting a Long Island case in which surgery was ordered to clear an intestinal blockage); Comment, "Defective Newborns: Inconsistent Application of Legal Principles Emphasized by Infant Doe Case," 14 Tex. Tech L. Rev. 569, 573 (1983) (reporting Detroit case); Shaw, "Dilemmas of 'Informed Consent' in Children," 289 New Eng. J. Med. 885, 887 (1973).

10. In re *McNulty*, No. 1960 (Prob. Ct. Essex County, Mass., Feb. 15, 1978), quoted in President's Commission, supra note 16, chapter 3, at 222 n.87; see also In re *Mueller*, No. 81J300 and 81J301 (5th Jud. Cir. Vermilion County, Ill., May 18, 1981) (surgery ordered to separate Siamese twins joined at the waist), noted in Shatten and Chabon, supra note 5.

11. *Custody of a Minor*, 434 N.E.2d 601, 604–605 (Mass. 1982).

12. In re *Guardianship of Barry*, 445 So.2d 365 (Fla. Dist. Ct. App. 1984).

13. The court record in the *Baby Doe* case was sealed. However, the case is discussed in detail in note, "Withholding Treatment from Defective Infants: 'Infant Doe' Postmortem," 59 Notre Dame L. Rev. 224, 225–235 (1983) and Longino, "Withholding Treatment from Defective Newborns: Who Decides, and on What Criteria," 31 U. Kans. L. Rev. 377 (1983).

14. See Diamond, supra note 37, chapter 2, at 56; Gustafson, "Mongolism, Parental Desires, and the Right to Life," 16 Perspectives in Biology and Med. 529 (1973) Shaw, supra note 9, at 887.

15. Shaw, Randolph and Manard, "Ethical Issues in Pediatric Surgery: A National Survey of Pediatricians and Pediatric Surgeons," 60 Pediatrics 588, 590 (1977). See also S. Rep. No. 246, 98th Cong., 1st Sess. 9 (1983) for a description of similar surveys of pediatricians' attitudes.

16. Duff and Campbell, "Moral and Ethical Dilemmas in the Special-Care Nursery," 289 New Eng. J. Med. 890, 891 (1973).

17. See Hauerwas, "Selecting Children to Live or Die: An Ethical Analysis of the Debate Between Dr. Lorber and Dr. Freeman on the Treatment of Meningomyelocele," in Death, Dying and Euthanasia, 228–247 (D. Horan & D. Mall, eds. 1977); Gross, Cox, et al. "Early Management and Decision-Making for the Treatment of Myelomeningocele," 72:4 Pediatrics 450, 452 (Oct. 1973).

18. See Shaw, Randolph & Manard, supra note 15.

19. See Fost, "Life and Death Decisions," in Rights and Responsibilities in Modern Medicine 57, 59–60 (Basson, ed. 1980); see also authorities listed in R. Wier, supra note 1.

20. American Academy of Pediatrics, Committee on Bioethics, "Treatment of Critically Ill Newborns," 72 Pediatrics 565, 566 (1983).

21. Current Opinions of the Judicial Council of the AMA § 2.10 (1982).

22. See generally *Who Speaks for the Child* (W. Gaylin and R. Macklin, eds. 1982); Goldstein, "Medical Care for the Child at Risk: On State Supervention of Parental Autonomy," 86 Yale L. J. 645 (1977); Shatten & Chabon, supra note 5.

23. Fleischman & Murray, "Ethics Committees for Infant Doe?," Hastings Cent. Rep., Dec. 1983, at 5; Diamond, supra note 37, chapter 2; Ellis, "Letting Defective Babies Die: Who Decides?," 7 Am. J.L. & Med. 393 (1982).

24. See Fletcher, "Attitudes Toward Defective Newborns," Hastings Cent. Rep., Jan. 1974, at 24–29.

25. Smith, "Life and Death Decisions in the Nursery," supra note 1 at 1132–1133; Note, "Withholding Treatment from Defective Infants," supra note (Fla. Dist. Ct. 1984); 13.

26. See In re *Guardianship of Barry*, 445 So.2d 365, 371–372; *Weber v. Stony Brook Hosp.*, 95 A.D.2d 587 (N.Y. App. Div.), modified, 456 N.E.2d 1186 (1983).

27. *Parham v. J.R.*, 442 U.S. 584, 602–603 (1979).

28. President's Commission, supra note 16, Chapter 3. See also Capron, "The Authority of Others to Decide about Biomedical Interventions with Incompetents," in Who Speaks for the Child 115–152 (W. Gaylin & R. Macklin, eds. 1982).

29. In re *Guardianship of Barry*, 445 So.2d 365.

30. See 45 C.F.R. § 84.55(f) (1984) (re Rehabilitation Act Regulations); 45 C.F.R. Part 1340, 49 Fed. Reg. 48162 (Dec. 10, 1984) (concerning regulations under the 1984 Child Care Amendments). Fost, "Baby Doe: Problems and Solutions," 1984 Ariz. St. L.J. 637 (discusses the advantages and hazards of infant care review committees).

31. See President's Commission, supra note 28, chapter 1, Fleischman and Murray, supra note 23. Not every commentator favors the use of an institutional ethics committee for decisions involving newborns. See Shatten and Chabon, supra note 5; Annas, "Baby Doe Redux: Doctors as Child Abusers," Hastings Cent. Rep., Oct. 1983, at 26.

32. Id. See also 49 Fed. Reg. 14900 (1985).

33. Id. at 14893, 14900.

34. AAP Infant Bioethics Task Force, supra note at 309; see also Annas, "Refusal of Lifesaving Treatment for Minors," 23 J. Fam. L. 217, 228 (1984–85).

35. Longino, supra note 13; Note, "Withholding Treatment from Defective Infants," supra note 13.

36. *Custody of a Minor*, 434 N.E.2d 601, 602–604.

37. *Weber v. Stony Brook Hosp.*, 456 N.E.2d 63, 65.

38. *Custody of a Minor*, 434 N.E.2d at 605; In re *Guardianship of Barry*, 445 So.2d at 371.

39. Macklin, "Return to the Best Interests of the Child," in Who Speaks for the Child 265, 290 (W. Gaylin and R. Macklin, eds. 1982); Smith, "Life and Death Decisions in the Nursery," supra note 1; R. Weir, supra note 1.

40. See *Custody of a Minor*, 379 N.E.2d 1053, 1063–1064; *Weber v. Stony Brook Hosp.*, 95 A.D.2d 587, 589; In re *Phillip B.*, 92 Cal. App. 3d 796, 803 (1979); Note, "Withholding Treatment from Defective Infants," supra note 13, (quoting from a letter received from the judge in the *Baby Doe* case in Indiana in 1982).

41. Current Opinions of the Judicial Council of the AMA § 2.10 (1982).

42. American Academy of Pediatrics, supra note 20.

43. President's Commission, supra note 28, chapter 1; R. Weir, supra note 1; Longino, supra note 13. A useful discussion of standards is found in Rhoden, "Treatment Decisions for Imperiled Newborns: Why Quality of Life Counts," 58 So. Calif. L. Rev. 1283 (1985).

44. See *People v. Labrenz*, 104 N.E.2d 769 (Ill. 1952); *Harrington v. State*, 547

S.W.2d 621 (Tex. Crim. App. 1977); Comment, "Defective Newborns," supra note 9.

45. R. Weir, supra note 1.

46. Id. at 236–237; Chapman and Goodall, "Helping a Child to Live Whilst Dying," 1980 The Lancet 753, 756; see also Morris, "Law, Morality, and Euthanasia for the Severely Defective Child," in Infanticide and the Value of Life 137, 147 (M. Kohl, ed. 1978). Congress, speaking to the issue of withholding of life-preserving care from infants, in the Child Abuse Amendments of 1984, noted that care should not be mandated where it would be "futile." See infra pp. 72–82 for discussion of this federal legislation.

47. *Custody of a Minor,* 434 N.E.2d at 609–610.

48. In re *Guardianship of Barry,* 445 So. 2d 365, 372.

49. See Feinberg and Ferry, "A Fate Worse Than Death: The Persistent Vegetative State in Childhood," 138 Am. J. Diseases Children 128–130 (1984).

50. Jonsen and Garland, "A Moral Policy for Life/Death Decisions in the Intensive Care Nursery," in Ethics of Newborn Intensive Care 142, 148 (A. Jonsen and M. Garland, eds. 1976).

51. In re *Daniels,* noted in Portela, supra note 8.

52. Strong, supra note 2; see President's Commission, supra note 16, chapter 3.

53. Strong, supra note 2; see Engelhardt, "Ethical Issues in Aiding the Death of Young Children," in Biomedical Ethics 384, 387–388 (T. Mappes and J. Zembaty, eds. 1981); Childress, "Triage in Neonatal Intensive Care: The Limitations of a Metaphor," 69 Va. L. Rev. 547, 558 (1983).

54. See Smith, "Life and Death Decisions in the Nursery," supra note 1; Koop, "Ethical and Surgical Considerations in the Care of the Newborn with Congenital Abnormalities," in Infanticide and the Handicapped Newborn 89–105 (D. Horan and M. Delahoyde, eds. 1982).

55. R. Weir, supra note 1, at 206. See also Cooke, "Whose Suffering?," 80 J. Pediatrics 906 (1972).

56. See Brandt, "Defective Newborns and the Morality of Termination," in Infanticide and the Value of Life 46, 49–50 (M. Kohl, ed. 1978); Longino, supra note 13.

57. The 1982 *Infant Doe* case, in which parents were permitted to decline surgical intervention for a Down's syndrome infant, was apparently argued and resolved on this basis of a prerogative to choose among various medical opinions. See Longino, supra note 13. Contra, In re *Daniels,* noted in Portela, supra note 8.

58. See generally Steinbock, "Baby Jane in the Courts," Hastings Cent. Rep., Feb. 1984, at 14, 18; *United States v. University Hosp.,* 729 F.2d 144 (2d Cir. 1984). There was conflicting information about just how impaired Baby Jane Doe's mental functioning was. One claim was that she had no upper brain function at all, but this was disputed. See Steinbock, supra at 14.

59. *Weber v. Stony Brook Hosp.,* 95 A.D. 2d 587.

60. Id. at 589.

61. See Barron, "Ruling Barring Surgery on Baby Won by Parents," *New York Times,* Oct. 22, 1983, at 26, col. 1; *Newark Star Ledger,* Nov. 5, 1983, at 6, col. 1; *New York Times,* April 7, 1984, at 28, col. 3.

62. HHS wanted to obtain the medical records of Baby Jane Doe in order to monitor the case, but the federal agency's efforts were rebuffed. See *United States v. University Hosp.,* 575 F. Supp. 607 (E.D.N.Y. 1983), aff'd, 729 F.2d 144. New York's highest state court upheld the Appellate Division's refusal to disrupt the parents' decision-making. That court's decision, though, was technically grounded on the inappropriateness of the petitioner—a private lawyer and right to life advocate—rather than on a full endorsement of the Appellate Division's rationale. *Weber v. Stony Brook Hosp.,* 456 N.E.2d 1186.

63. See Goldstein, supra note 22, at 664. Also found in Who Speaks for the Child 153, 178–179 (W. Gaylin and R. Macklin, eds. 1982).

64. Juvenile Justice Standards Project, ABA-Institute of Judicial Administration, Abuse and Neglect 73–74 (1981); In re *Jensen,* 633 P.2d 1302 (Or. Ct. App. 1981).

65. Id. See also R. Veatch, *Death, Dying, and the Biological Revolution,* (Yale 1976), at 125–127.

66. See In re *Hofbauer,* 393 N.E.2d 1009 (N.Y. 1979).

67. See R. Veatch, supra note 65; Juvenile Justice Standards Project, supra note 64; Macklin, supra note 39; Sokolosky, "The Sick Child and the Reluctant Parent—A Framework for Judicial Intervention," 20 J. Fam. L. 69, 76–81 (1981–1982).

68. See In re *Philip B.,* 92 Cal. App. 3d 796; In re *Hudson,* 126 P. 765 (Wash. 1942); In re *Seiferth,* 127 N.E.2d 820 (N.Y. 1955); In re *Tuttendario,* 21 Pa. D. 561 (1912).

69. In re *Hofbauer,* 393 N.E.2d 1009, 1013–1014; see Note, "The Outer Limits of Parental Autonomy: Withholding Medical Treatment from Children," 42 Ohio St. L.J. 813, 817–820 (1981). Parents can not only decline medical intervention because of toxic or fatal risks, but they can authorize somewhat risky procedures in an effort to improve the quality of life of a child. For example, in October 1983 parents of the Houston "Bubble Boy"—a twelve year old with immune deficiency who had lived for years isolated in a plastic coated world— took the risk of a bone marrow transplant in the hope of freeing the lad from the bubble world. The operation failed and the boy died in February 1984. But no one suggested that the parents were neglectful for having subjected their son to a fatal risk. See *Newark Star Ledger,* Feb.16, 1984, at 47, col. 1; Smith, supra note 1.

70. See In re *Jensen,* 633 P.2d 1302, 1306; *Application of Cicero,* 101 Misc. 2d 699.

71. See *Custody of a Minor,* 379 N.E.2d 1053, 1063–1064; In re *Daniels,* noted in Portela, supra note 8.

72. See Sokolosky, supra note 67.

73. *United States v. University Hosp.,* 729 F.2d at 146.

74. Steinbock, supra note 58.

75. On the "Johns Hopkins" case, see Gustafson, supra note 14, at 529–557; Freeman, "The 'God Committee'," *New York Times,* May 21, 1972, at 84 § 6 (magazine), col. 4. See also Longino, supra note 13, at 388–389, and Annas, "Denying the Rights of the Retarded: The Philip Becker Case," Hastings Cent. Rep., Dec. 1979, at 18–20, describing how the needs of "the rest of the family" played a role in rejecting life-prolonging treatment for a twelve-year-old Down's syndrome child in the case of In re *Philip B.,* 92 Cal. App. 3d 796.

76. Gross, Cox et al., "Early Management and Decision-Making for the Treatment of Myelomeningocele," 72:4 Pediatrics (Oct. 1973), p. 454.

77. Shaw, Randolph and Manard, supra note 15.

78. Cobrinik, "Decisions for the Defective Newborn," 11, 13 in Life and Death Decisions (A. Winter, ed. 1980); Brandt, supra note 56.

79. See, e.g., Shatten & Chabon, supra note 5; Brandt, supra note 56, at 55; Strong, supra note 2; R. Weir, supra note 1.

80. R. Weir, supra note 1, at 214–215. See also Strong, supra note 2; Engelhardt, supra note 53.

81. See Garland, "Views on the Ethics of Infant Euthanasia," in Ethics of Newborn Intensive Care 126, 127 (A. Jonsen and M. Garland, eds. 1976).

82. Strong, supra note 2, at 14.

83. See, e.g., *Jefferson v. Griffin Spalding County Hosp. Auth.,* 274 S.E.2d 457, 459 (Ga. 1981); 18 Pa. Cons. Stat. Ann. § 3212 (Purdon 1983).

84. One glaring exception may be the *Infant Doe* case in Indiana in 1982 in which the court refused to overturn a parental refusal to authorize life-preserving surgery for a mongoloid child. The record in the case was sealed and the relevant court opinions were not published, making it impossible to know the extent to which the Indiana courts allowed family interests to be weighed in the decision-making process.

85. See, e.g., President's Commission, supra note 28, chapter 1; Annas, "Disconnecting the Baby Doe Hotline," Hastings Cent. Rep., June 1983, at 15; Smith, "Life and Death Decisions in the Nursery," supra note 1.

86. Current Opinions of the Judicial Council of the AMA § 2.10 (1982).

87. AAP, Official Policy on Treatment of Critically Ill Newborns, 72:4 Pediatrics (Oct 1983), p. 566.

88. N.Y. Fam. Ct. Act § 1012(f)(i)(A) (Consol. 1981). See also So. Car. Stat. § 20-7-490(c)(3)(1976); R. I. Stat. § 40-11-2(2)(d)(1984 Supp.); W. Va. Stat. § 49-1-3(1) (1984 Supp.).

89. See McCarthy, Koops, Honeyfield & Butterfield, "Who Pays the Bill for Neonatal Intensive Care?," 95 J. Pediatrics 755, 755–761 (1979).

90. See Goldstein, supra note 22. Professor Goldstein also insists that government must provide suitable adopting parents if the natural parents choose not to care for a defective newborn. For a similar approach, emphasizing a state "obligation" to provide for the special needs of handicapped children, see President's Commission, supra note 28, chapter 1, at 229. See also note, "Withholding Treatment from Defective Infants," supra note 13.

91. R. Weir, supra note 164 at 196. However, Professor Weir would allow family interests to influence decision-making for defective newborns at least in exceptional cases. Id. at 258-260.

92. *Roe v. Wade*, 410 U.S. 113, 163–164 (1973).

93. See, e.g., La. Rev. Stat. Ann. § 40:1299.36.2(A) (West Supp. 1985); Unif. Adoption Act § 19, 9 U.L.A. 51 (1985); Juvenile Justice Standards Project, supra note 64.

94. See Robertson, "Procreative Liberty and the Control of Conception, Pregnancy, and Childbirth," 69 Va. L. Rev. 405, 458–462 (1983).

95. Goldstein, supra note 22; Duff and Campbell, supra note 16.

96. Smith, "On Letting Some Babies Die," Hastings Cent. Rep., May 1974, at 45.

97. These figures are drawn from Strong, supra note 2.

98. See Rosenblum and Budde, "Historical and Cultural Considerations of Infanticide," in Infanticide and the Handicapped Newborn 11 (D. Horan & M. Delahoyde, eds. 1982); R. Weir, supra note 1.

99. See Kramer, "Ethical Issues in Neonatal Intensive Care: An Economic Perspective," in Ethics of Newborn Intensive Care 75, 89–91 (A. Jonsen & M. Garland, eds. 1976).

100. Hodgman, "Withholding Treatment from Seriously Ill Newborns: A Neonatologist's View," in Legal and Ethical Aspects of Treating Critically and Terminally Ill Patients 242, 245 (A. Doudera & J. Peters, eds. 1982).

101. Levinson, Book Review, 96 Harv. L. Rev. 1466, 1483 (1983). See also Margolis, "Human Life: Its Worth and Bringing it to an End," in Infanticide and the Value of Life 180, 189 (M. Kohl, ed. 1978).

102. See Comment, "Defective Newborns," supra note 9; Koop, supra note 54.

103. The judge in the *Infant Doe* case in Indiana is quoted as relying in part on "the family's right to be free from undue government interference." note, "Withholding Treatment from Defective Infants," supra note 13. See also In re *Guardianship of Barry*, 445 So. 2d 365; *Weber v. Stony Brook Hosp.*, 456 N.E.2d 1186, 1188.

104. *Santosky v. Kramer,* 455 U.S. 745, 753 (1982).

105. See *Parham v. J.R.,* 442 U.S. 584, 602; *Lehr v. Robertson,* 463 U.S. 248, 257–258 (1983); *Halderman v. Pennhurst State School & Hosp.,* 707 F.2d 702, 706 (3d Cir. 1983); see Olsen, "The Family and the Market: A Study of Ideology and Legal Reform," 96 Harv. L. Rev. 1497, 1505 (1983).

106. See *Lehr v. Robertson,* 463 U.S. 248, 256–257; *Quillion v. Walcott,* 434 U.S. 246 (1978).

107. *Parham v. J.R.,* 442 U.S. 584, 604.

108. See In re *Grady,* 426 A.2d 467, 475, 482.

109. See, e.g., *Jehovah's Witnesses v. King County Hosp.,* 278 F. Supp. 488 (W.D. Wash. 1967), aff'd, 390 U.S. 598 (1968); *State v. Clark,* 261 A.2d 294, 300 (Conn. Cir. Ct. 1969); Macklin, supra note 39; Bennett, "Allocation of Child Medical Care Decision-Making Authority: A Suggested Interest Analysis," 62 U. Va. L. Rev. 285, 323–324 (1976). Sometimes, pregnant mothers have been ordered to undergo medical procedures in order to protect the potential infant being carried to term. See *Raleigh Fitkin-Paul Morgan Mem. Hosp. v. Anderson,* 201 A.2d 537 (N.J. 1964) (blood transfusion); *Jefferson v. Griffin Spalding County Hosp. Auth.,* 274 S.E.2d 457 (caesarean section).

110. See Va. Code § 18.2-371.1 (1982); Juvenile Justice Standards Project, supra note 64.

111. See *Application of Cicero,* 101 Misc. 2d 699; In re *Jensen,* 633 P.2d 1302, 1305.

112. See *Halderman v. Pennhurst State School & Hosp.,* 707 F.2d 702, 712-715 (Rosenn, Circuit Judge, concurring); Robertson, supra note 94; Sokolosky, supra note 67.

113. See President's Commission, supra note 28, chapter 1; Capron, supra note 28; Veatch, "The Technical Criteria Fallacy," Hastings Cent. Rep., Aug. 1977, at 15.

114. See In re *Philip B.,* 92 Cal. App. 3d 796, 802; *State v. Clark,* 261 A.2d 294, 298; Note, "Withholding Treatment from Defective Infants," supra note 13, quoting the judge who rendered the *Infant Doe* decision in Indiana in 1982.

115. 29 U.S.C. § 794 (1982). For extensive discussion of Section 504, see Vitiello, "The Baby Jane Doe Litigation and Section 504: An Exercise in Raw Executive Power," 17 Conn. L. Rev. 95 (1984); see also Mathieu, "The Baby Doe Controversy," 1984 Ariz. St. L.J. 605, 606–612; and Note, "Defective Newborns and Section 504 of the Rehabilitation Act: Legislation by Administrative Fiat?," 25 Ariz. L. Rev. 709 (1983).

116. Notice to Health Care Providers, 47 Fed. Reg. 26,027 (1982).

117. See Vitiello, supra note 115; Note, "Defective Newborns and Section 504," supra note 115; *United States v. University Hosp.,* 729 F.2d 144, 156.

118. 47 Fed. Reg. 26,027 (1982).

119. 48 Fed. Reg. 9630 (1983) (to be codified at 45 C.F.R. pt. 84) (interim final rule approved Mar. 2, 1983).

120. *American Academy Pediatrics v. Heckler,* 561 F. Supp. 395 (D.D.C. 1983).

121. 48 Fed. Reg. 30,846 (1983) (to be codified at 45 C.F.R. pt. 84) (modifying 84 C.F.R. pt. 84.61).

122. 49 Fed. Reg. 1622 (1984) (to be codified at 45 C.F.R. pt. 84) (effective Feb. 13, 1984).

123. 49 Fed. Reg. 1654 (1984). See Annas, "Refusal of Lifesaving Treatment for Minors," 23 J. Fam. L. 217, 226 (1984–85).

124. For a summary of the criticisms of the HHS Baby Doe Regulations, see Mathieu, supra note 115; Meyer, supra note 2. HHS itself has summarized some of the criticisms which its tentative regulations received. See 49 Fed. Reg. 1622–1654.

125. The first ruling against the revised HHS regulations came in the context of federal litigation relating to the *Baby Jane Doe* case decided in New York state courts in 1983. The New York state courts had refused to disrupt the parental decision not to authorize surgery for their infant daughter suffering from spina bifida. See note, "Withholding Treatment from Defective Infants," supra note 13. In February 1984, the Federal Second Circuit Court of Appeals repudiated an HHS effort to get access to Baby Jane Doe's medical records. In that ruling, the court found the proposed HHS regulations to be unauthorized by Congress. See *United States v. University Hosp.*, 729 F.2d 144. The American Hospital Association (AHA) then relied on that ruling to successfully attack the revised HHS regulations. See *American Hosp. Assoc. v. Heckler*, 585 F. Supp. 541 (S.D.N.Y. 1984), aff'd, (2d Cir. 1984) (unpublished opinion), cert. granted 53 U.S.L.W. 387 (U.S. June 18, 1985) (No. 84-1529).

126. *Southeastern Community College v. Davis*, 442 U.S. 397 (1979); *Doe v. New York Univ.*, 666 F.2d 761 (2d Cir. 1981).

127. See 49 Fed. Reg. 1630, 1653.

128. Id. at 1653.

129. See S. Rep. No. 246, 98th Cong., 2d Sess. 9 (1984). However, the Surgeon General has also been quoted as saying that the regulations do not require preservation of an infant born without a digestive tract even though such an infant might be maintained for up to eighteen months. See 73 Pediatrics 262 (1984); Note, "Withholding Treatment from Birth-Defective Newborns: The Search for an Elusive Standard," 31 Wayne L. Rev. 187, 204 n.101 (1984).

130. 130 Cong. Rec. H 382–383 (1984); 130 Cong. Rec. S 9311 (1984) (letter from the National Right to Life Committee).

131. 130 Cong. Rec. S 12,392 (1984) (Letter from the six leading Senate sponsors of the bill relating to medical care for defective newborns).

132. Pub. L. No. 98-457, Title I, §§ 122, 128, 128(b), 98 Stat. 1752, 1755 (1984). For a review of the legislation as it relates to defective newborns, see note, "The Child Abuse Amendments of 1984: The Infant Doe Amendment," 18 Akron L. Rev. 515 (1985).

133. See H.R. Rep. No. 1038, 98th Cong., 2d Sess. 26 (1984); 130 Cong. Rec. S9313 (1984).

134. See H.R. Rep. No. 1038, 98th Cong., 2d Sess. 24 (1984); 130 Cong. Rec. S9318, S9320 (1984).

135. H.R. Rep. No. 1038, 98th Cong., 2d Sess. 43 (1984).

136. See Pub. L. No. 98-457, Title I, § 201(a), discussed at 130 Cong. Rec. H 10,329, H 10,333, S9318.

137. 130 Cong. Rec. H 10,327 (1984) (Rep. Murphy); 130 Cong. Rec. S9320 (1984) (Sen. Dodd); see also 130 Cong. Rec. S12,392.

138. See list of federal involvements in "Baby Doe" investigations supplied by HHS as part of its final "Baby Doe" regulations. 49 Fed. Reg. 1622, 1642–1643, 1646–1649 (1984).

139. Pub. L. No. 98-457, Title I, § 121(3), 98 Stat. 1752 (1984).

140. 130 Cong. Rec. S12,383, S12,385, H 10,330-331 (1984).

141. See 130 Cong. Rec. H399-400, S9321 (1984).

142. 130 Cong. Rec. H392-398 (1984).

143. See Vitiello, supra note 115; Rhoden, supra note 43, at 1313–17.

144. See 49 Fed. Reg. 48160, et seq. (1984).

145. 49 Fed. Reg. 48164, 48167 (1984).

146. Id. at 48167.

147. Id. at 48164, 48167.

148. See 50 Fed. Reg. 14879 (1985).

149. Id. at 14880, 14889.

150. Id. at 14880, 14890, 14892.
151. Id. at 14892.
152. 130 Cong. Rec. S9319 (1984).
153. 130 Cong. Rec. S9324 (1984). One commentator has suggested that "virtually futile" means that life cannot be preserved for an extended period, perhaps beyond a year or two. Vitiello, supra note 115, at 156–157. This is a possible interpretation, but would only make sense if "futile" in the prior statutory exception were confined to situations in which death is fairly imminent, i.e., where further treatment will immediately be futile. The statutory intention, as indicated in the letter from six legislative sponsors, seems otherwise.
154. See notes 86 and 87, supra.
155. See note 152 supra.
156. Murray, "The Final, Anticlimactic Rule on Baby Doe," 15:3 Hastings Cent. Rep., June 1985, at 9.
157. 50 Fed. Reg. 14884 (1985).
158. Murray, supra note 156, at 6.
159. The 1985 regulations issued by HHS comment: "The Department believes that these interpretive guidelines [the Appendix to the regulations] can and should be referred to by interested parties in understanding, interpreting, and applying the statutory definitions." HHS also pointed out that HHS is the agency charged with implementation of the statute. 50 Fed. Reg. 14882 (1985).
160. See pp. 142–43, infra, for the specifics of recent state legislation on this subject.
161. See 130 Cong. Rec. H384-385; 50 Fed. Reg. 14892 (1985).
162. 1982 La. Acts 339, codified at La. Rev. Stat. Ann. § 40:1299.36.1(B) (West Supp. 1985).
163. La. Rev. Stat. Ann. § 40:1299.36.1(C), (D) (West Supp. 1985).
164. Id. at 1299.36.1(A).
165. Ariz. Rev. Stat. Ann. § 36-2281.(A) (Supp. 1975–1984).
166. Id. at 2281.(D).
167. Id. at 2281.(C)(3).
168. Id. at 2281.(C)(2).
169. Ariz. Rev. Stat. Ann. § 36-2284(A), (B) (Supp. 1975–1984). For commentary on the 1984 Arizona legislation, see Mathieu, supra note 115.
170. Ariz. Rev. Stat. Ann. § 36-2281(A) (Supp. 1975–1984).
171. Ind. Code Ann. § 31-6-4-3(f) (West Supp. 1985).
172. See Mnookin, "Two Puzzles," 1984 Ariz. St. L.J. 667, 668, 677–679; Mathieu, supra note 115; R. Wier, supra note 1.
173. For a particularly graphic description of the progressive deterioration accompanying a starvation process, see *Brophy*, supra, slip opinion at pp. 28–29.
174. See, e.g., Smith, "Life and Death Decisions in the Nursery: Standards and Procedures for Withholding Lifesaving Treatment from Infants," 27 N.Y. L. Rev. 1125, 1169 (1982); Cobrinik, supra note 78 at 16; Note, "The Outer Limits of Parental Autonomy: Withholding Medical Treatment from Children," 42 Ohio State L.J. 813, 829 (1981).
175. See pp. 78–82, chapter 3. See also Rhoden, supra note 43.

Chapter VII: Afterword: On Death and the Quality of Life

1. 50 Fed. Reg. 14889 (1985).
2. Even Professor Robert Burt, a staunch opponent of a broad prerogative to withhold life-preserving care from infants, concedes that in extreme cases the avoidance of suffering warrants the allowance of death. See Burt, "The Ideal of

Community in the Work of the President's Commission," 6 Cardozo L. Rev. 267, 284 (1984).

3. See *Procanik v. Cillo*, 478 A.2d 755 (N.J. 1984).

4. Public L. No. 98-457, Title I, #121(3), 98 Stat. 1752 (1984); see commentary in Rhoden, supra note 43, chapter 6.

5. "Ethics of Newborn Intensive Care" (Jonsen and Garland, eds. 1976), pp. 143–44.

INDEX

Alzheimers' disease: imminence of death, 14; withdrawal of nutrition, 100; court approval of do not resuscitate orders, 104

American Academy of Pediatrics: survey of physicians' views on nontreatment of infants, 128, 130; ethics committees, 132, 133, 134; "best interests" standard, 137, 148; sued to prevent implementation of 1984 Health and Human Services regulations, 157; endorsed Child Abuse Amendments of 1984, 165; approval of 1985 Health and Human Services regulations, 169–70

American Hospital Association: sued to prevent implementation of Health and Human Services regulations, 157, 159; endorsed Child Abuse Amendments of 1984, 165

American Medical Association: economic factors, 89, 91; CPR inappropriate in terminal cases, 104; endorsed decision-making authority of family and physician, 118; parental choice for defective infants, 130; endorsed "best interests" standard for infants, 136–37, 148; opposed Child Abuse Amendments of 1984, 165

American Nurses' Association: endorsed Child Abuse Amendments of 1984, 165

Arizona state legislature: prohibition of nontreatment of infants, 170–72

Arkansas state legislature: approval of terminal decisions without judicial involvement, 115

Association for Retarded Citizens: endorsed Child Abuse Amendments of 1984, 165

Baby Jane Doe case: controversy, 128; conservative medical approach selected by parents, 141–43, 144–45, 168

Bambrick, Justice: decision on physician's liability, 18

Barber v. Superior Court: omission vs. commission in treatment of terminal patients, 32; active termination of treatment, 33; nutrition as medical procedure, 41–42

Bartling: hospital refusal to halt treatment, 11, 188n; nonimminence of death, 55

Bludworth: decision left to family and physicians, 118; value as precedent unclear, 194n

Bouvia v. Riverside Hospital: hunger strike by handicapped disallowed, 28–30; rejection of nutrition as suicide, 51, 52

Bowen v. American Hospital Association: application of Rehabilitation Act of 1973 to infants not authorized by Congress, 158–59

Brooks Estate: religious principles, 22

Brophy v. New England Sinai Hospital: hospital refusal to withdraw artificial nutrition, 101–103, 189n

Burt, Robert: witholding of treatment from infants in extreme cases, 202n

California Natural Death Act, 7–8

California state courts: competent patient's right to reject treatment, 11; overruled hunger strike by handicapped, 28–29; "extraordinary" treatment dichotomy, 37–38; nutrition viewed as medical procedure, 41–42, 43; rejection of nutrition as suicide, 51, 52; terminal decisions without judicial involvement approved, 114

California state legislature: Natural Death Act, 7–8; appointment of proxy for terminal decision-making, 123

Callahan, Daniel: nutrition as a symbol, 39

Campbell, Doctor: report on infant deaths, 129

Capron, Alexander: counterproductivity of judicial intervention in terminal decisions, 115

Catholic theology: influence on courts, 35–36; nutrition not a medical treatment, 38; rejection of treatment not suicide, 48; economic considerations, 89–90

Chemotherapy: rejection of in nonimminent cases, 13; mentally handicapped patients, 92

Child abuse: parental responsibility to infant, 147–48; fiscal burden defense, 148–49, 151; statutory limits on parental au-

NORMAN L. CANTOR, senior faculty member at Rutgers University School of Law, Newark, N.J., and a visiting professor at Tel Aviv University's Faculty of Law, is author of a number of law journal articles on the legal aspects of death and dying.